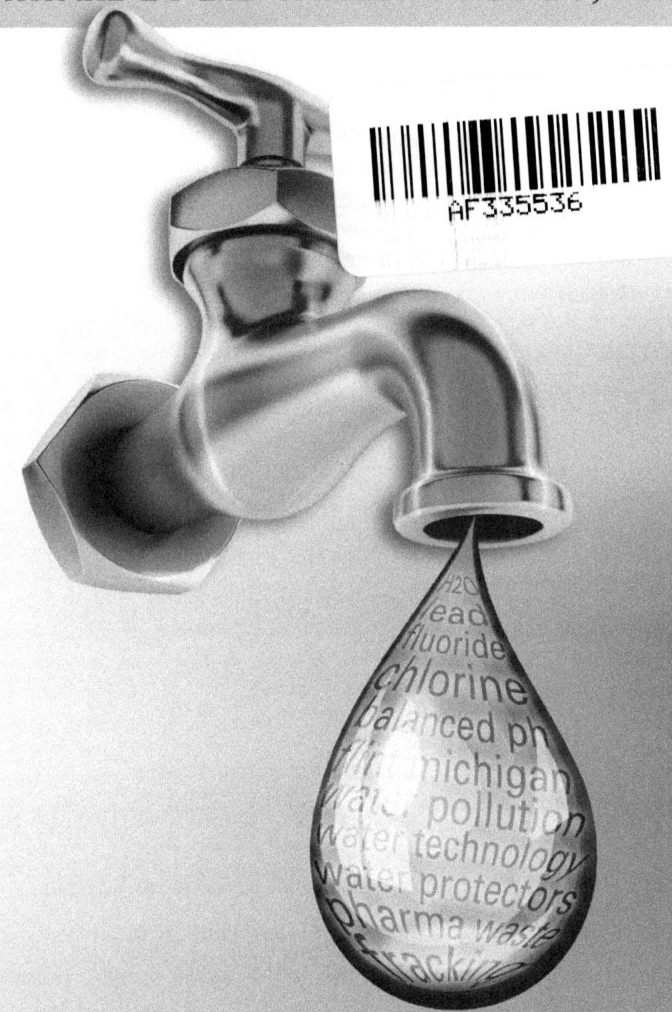

THE RACE TO PROTECT OUR MOST IMPORTANT NATURAL RESOURCE:

WATER

SAMUEL K. BURLUM

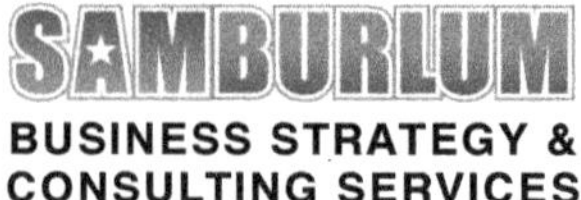

**BUSINESS STRATEGY &
CONSULTING SERVICES**

www.samburlum.com

Library of Congress Cataloging -in- Publication Data - Burlum, Sam

The Race to Protect Our Most Important Natural Resource: Water

ISBN: 978-0-9988872-0-3 (softcover)

Cover Art: Brand Worx Productions

Layout: Lloyd Arbour

Editor: Lucille Pearce

Consultant: Dan Hollis, The Magic of Selling

First published 2017

Copyright © 2017 Sam Burlum

Quantity discounts are available on bulk orders.
Contact samburlum@gmail.com for more information.

DEDICATION

I dedicate this work to those who have committed their lives and their work's purpose to uplifting our human family, in advocating for access to clean, fresh, drinking water for all people, even when profit dictates otherwise.

A portion of the proceeds from the sales of this book will be dedicated and donated to non-profit causes that are helping communities and villages gain access to clean, fresh, drinking water by establishing community freshwater wells and pump stations. These non-profit causes also educate and train members within the community on how to maintain the equipment and the quality of water. Best practices are adopted in preserving and protecting the new resource.

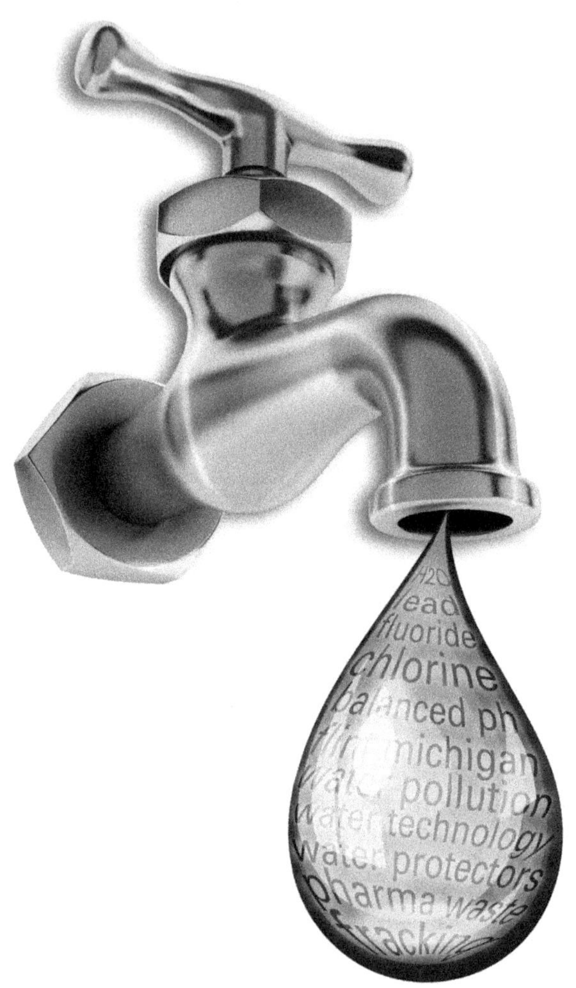

H2O
lead
fluoride
chlorine
balanced ph
flint michigan
water pollution
water technology
water protectors
pharma waste
fracking

TABLE OF CONTENTS:

Disclaimer 7

Acknowledgements 9

Forward by Dr. Carley Corrado 11

Introduction 15

Chapter 1: Source of the Problem 21

Chapter 2: Distribution and Delivery 27

Chapter 3: Quantity Versus Quality. 33

Chapter 4: So What's in Your Water?. 39

Chapter 5: Where Does the Best Water Come From?. 47

Chapter 6: The Most Endangered Fresh Drinking
Water Sources in the World 53

Chapter 7: The Real Cost/Price for Quality Drinking Water 61

Chapter 8: You are What You Drink 67

Chapter 9: The Importance of a pH Balanced Water 73

Chapter 10: Putting Water to Work for You 79

Chapter 11: Water's Other Valuable Roles in our
Modern Society. 85

Chapter 12: New Technology Aimed At Reducing Water Usage. . . 93

Chapter 13: Battles on the Waterfront; Where Environment,
Industry, and Public Policy Clash 101

Chapter 14: New Public Policies at Work in Protecting
Drinking Water Sources 109

Chapter 15: Methods for Testing the Quality of Water at Home. . 117

Chapter 16: Remediation Ideas for at Home 125

Chapter 17: Water Preservation and Conservation
Tips for Use at Home. 133

Appendix:

Cited Resources 139

Glossary. 149

About the Author 155

DISCLAIMER

In a time of rapid change it is difficult to ensure that all of the information in this book is entirely accurate and current. This publication is designed to provide accurate and authoritative information. The author specifically disclaims any liability, loss or risk, personal or otherwise, which anyone may incur as a consequence of the use and application of any of the contents of this book.

The information contained herein is a collection of research, which is sited from other sources, and should not be reviewed as medical or legal advice. The opinions and comments provided, referenced from interviews, may not be the direct opinion or position of this author.

When investigating technology or chemical remedies, the reader is advised to abide by the manufacturer's recommendations and/or instructions and cautionary disclaimers within owner's guides and/or Safety Data Sheets.

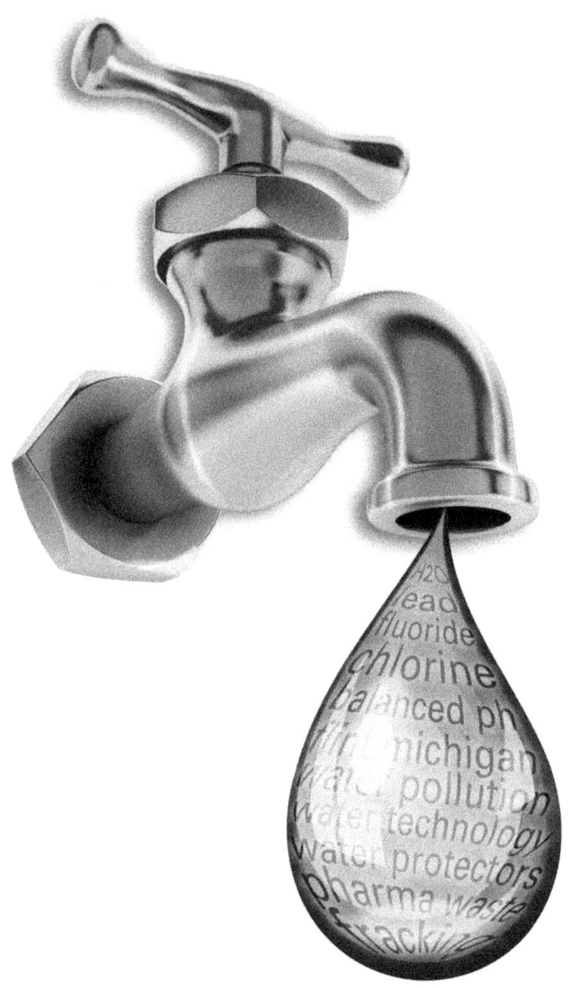
H2O
lead
fluoride
chlorine
balanced ph
michigan
water pollution
water technology
water protectors
pharma waste
fracking

ACKNOWLEDGEMENTS

I want to thank all who contributed to the content of this book. Their participation in providing information and perspectives was critical in conveying the bigger picture of protecting our most important natural resource, water.

I also want to thank those who search for ways to provide clean, fresh, drinking water to impoverished communities that cannot afford pure, uncontaminated, consumable water. Your leadership and commitment in uplifting villages and communities through education and the installation of new community water wells and pump stations have changed those lives forever for generations to come. Those who had an uncertain future now have hope for a brighter tomorrow.

I would like to thank the water protectors for their continued efforts informing residents and citizens about industry and public policy debates which impact clean drinking water. These groups include non-profit organizations and individuals that bring awareness through educational platforms, articles, and community events.

There is a group of water protectors made up of private citizens of this nation and other nations that have taken a peaceful stand against profit when it destroys planet and people. We thank you for taking time out to stand up for our most important natural resource.

I want to thank many of the eco-boomer generation who are living the life of environmental sustainability. Their lifestyle and consumer choices have begun to shape policy and provoke open conversations about this critical societal issue. These younger generations are voting with their consumer dollars. They are reversing policies that generations before them have neglected to correct. Many of these young individuals are now putting their skill sets to work in order to usher in new methods and technology aimed at solving these problems.

FORWARD

Water is truly at the core of life on this planet. Water is the major constituent of the human body, as well as the surface of the Earth. Hence, it is not a huge leap to say that the health of our water is inextricably linked to the health of our bodies, our society, and the flourishing of all of life.

In this book, *The Race to Protect the Most Important Natural Resource: Water*, Samuel K. Burlum provides an excellent brief and well-rounded look on the issues surrounding water today.

The current challenge of having enough clean water is vast and intimidating. The issues are broken down into concise explanations with tangible instructions on how to address the challenges.

The purpose of this book is to encourage *empowerment*. The reader is informed of current issues broken down into simple terms and given instructions as to what actions to take.

It will explain how to test your water, what type of filtration may be needed and how to be an educated consumer of water. Additional great resources are provided for any issue needing further explanation.

This book is informative for readers who hope to become knowledgeable about local issues surrounding their own water supply. Since water everywhere needs advocacy, this guide provides the information necessary for a concerned citizen to start asking pertinent questions and take action.

Despite the challenges that lie ahead, new technologies are being developed every day with improved designs that work with nature rather than against it. In addition, new policies are being put in place to protect the environment and hence ultimately humanity. While pressure from industry appears to be increasing the pollution and toxicity of the world, history has taught us the power of regulation to shift industrial practices to be harmonious with life and the health of generations to come.

Before the Environmental Protector Agency (EPA) was established, air pollution and toxic dumping were the norm. With pressure from the public, legislators introduced the Clear Air Act of 1970, the Pesticide Control Act of 1972, the Ocean Dumping Act of 1972, and the Safe Drinking Water Act of 1974, to mention a few. There are photos from our own country's history showing air pollution as bad as Beijing, China, with waterways loaded with dumped vehicles and trash.

Our country's environmental safety is surprisingly better than it has been in the past. However, we are not yet currently where we need to be as a society in terms of the plentitude of clean water for drinking, agriculture, industry, and a healthy ecosystems. The past has shown us the power that we have when we use our minds to develop innovative solutions and use our voices to insure that the policy-makers regulate industry, agriculture, and land use in order to preserve and even improve the health of our society for many generations to come.

We can impact our future by understanding the challenges of today. *The Race to Protect the Most Important Natural Resource: Water* is a great place to be informed. It is full to the brim with relevant information, yet written in a very concise and simplified way. Cheers to a great read!

— Dr. Carley Corrado, PhD
Renewable Energy and Soil Scientist

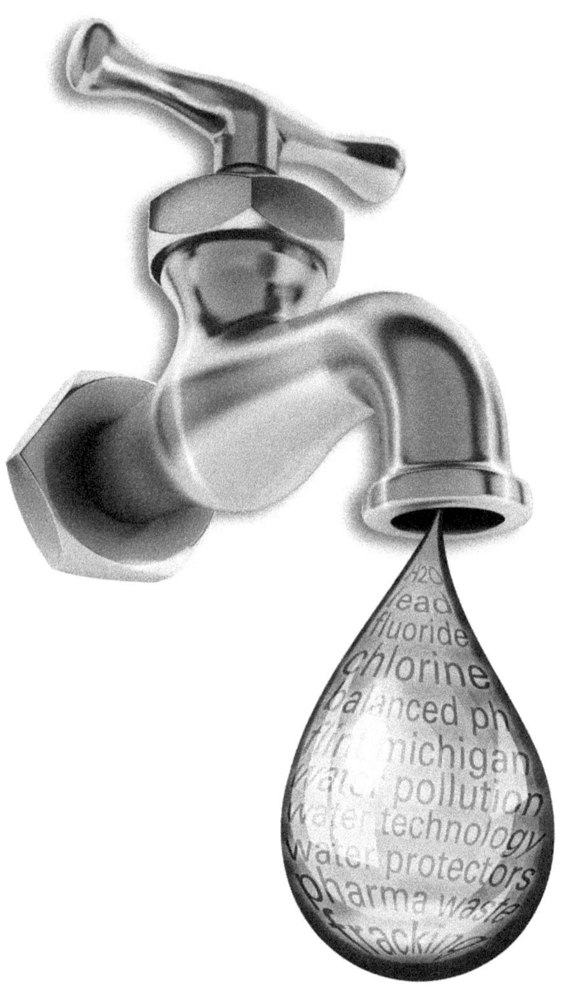

H2O
lead
fluoride
chlorine
balanced ph
flint michigan
water pollution
water technology
water protectors
pharma waste
fracking

INTRODUCTION

What is in your water? Do you really know how safe your drinking water is? Do you trust where it comes from?

Residents of Flint, Michigan thought they had a trusted water source, but the growing issues of aging infrastructure, polluted water sources, and chemical invasion, over time developed into a disastrous combination, creating a negative effect on its city's population.

In our fast paced society, necessities that we appreciated hundreds of years ago, are often now taken for granted. We fail to do our due diligence in having a comprehensive understanding of the adverse issues concerning water; our most important natural resource.

Education on this subject matter is vital, as it directly affects our personal health, our ability to sustain a healthy and vibrant community, as well as experience a fruitful economy. Without water, we as a species would cease to exist.

Flint, Michigan is only one example of how communities around the world are trying to cope with the critical issues of tainted drinking water supplies or the disappearance of clean, fresh, drinking water all together.

Water has been referred to as the next "blue gold." I address issues of concerns in this book so that we can have a better understanding the following:

a. What exactly is in our water?

b. How can we mitigate the hazards?

c. How does the quality of the water affect our health?

d. What are the most threatened water sources on our planet?

e. How can YOU help in preserving our most important natural resource?

These discussion points and more are aimed to raise awareness of the bigger issues at stake, with suggestions and remedies on how we can take a personal approach to help solve these challenges.

Let us take a moment to examine issues that exist in our own back yard. Then, from a 10,000-foot view above, we can compare those challenges to examples of what has happened around the world in regions where the seriousness of water quality has resulted in consequences of such magnitude that some communities and economies have been destroyed.

In discussing the current state of affairs of clean, fresh drinking water, I provide a panoramic view of the business of the water industry, the public policy that influences it and the real cost to consumers for their supply of clean, fresh, drinking water. I present a financial, as well as a health and wellness perspective.

You will learn about key debates now affecting future supplies of clean, fresh, drinking water and how you can influence the outcomes of public policy in areas of water quality and preservation.

You will also learn about cost-effective steps to take in order to conserve water, starting in your own home. You will discover how to remove influences that rob us daily of clean, fresh, drinking water.

Finally, I am hoping this book will bring you a new awareness on how one's own personal choices affect the rest of the planet and its population. You will understand the cumulative effect each person's individual attitude and actions has on this most important natural resource.

When I was hired as a business consultant for a bottled water company, I was not well educated about the real issues that plague the industry. I was unaware of the entire dynamic in play between an industry that profits from a consumable, which seems to me to be one of those God given rights, and the disconnect from those individuals and communities that only dream of having clean, fresh, drinking water.

I became increasingly interested in having a greater understanding of how my influence as a business leader could either help or hurt the industry. Thus, through this book, I sought to use my leadership role on a new level to assist in solving some of these challenges. It is my hope that individuals that do not yet have access to fresh, clean drinking water, may be granted this very essence to our existence.

As I dug deep into the research, putting all the puzzle pieces together, it became apparent that I had an obligation to share the information contained in this book to help others become educated and aware of these matters. It is my intent to encourage us to take personal responsibility for our consumption of water, play a role in preserving the limited sources of water that our planet supplies, and help others obtain this vital resource where fresh, clean drinking water is viewed as a luxury.

I invite you to read through this collection of research notes, interviews, facts and tips on how to play your part to insure a positive outcome for our society's current challenges to best preserve our natural water sources.

Please take notice of the following mentioned chapters. I hope to give you a greater understanding on how you can protect your family from tainted water sources and how you can recognize them. I provide you remedies and methods to consider adopting to mitigate bad water at the tap.

In Chapter Four, you will get a list of all the potential chemicals found in your drinking water source.

Chapter Seven takes a view of the real cost of quality, clean, fresh drinking water.

Chapter Eight discusses the influence water quality may have on the human body.

Chapter Fifteen explains how you can test the water that comes out of your faucet.

Chapters Sixteen and Seventeen outline a host of technologies, products and practices aimed at mitigating water quality issues. You will learn how you can play a part in conserving water supplies.

I invite you to read this entire work to fully understand why we must take a new approach to protect our most important natural resource, why it is critical, and why each of us has a role in preserving clean, fresh drinking water for future generations.

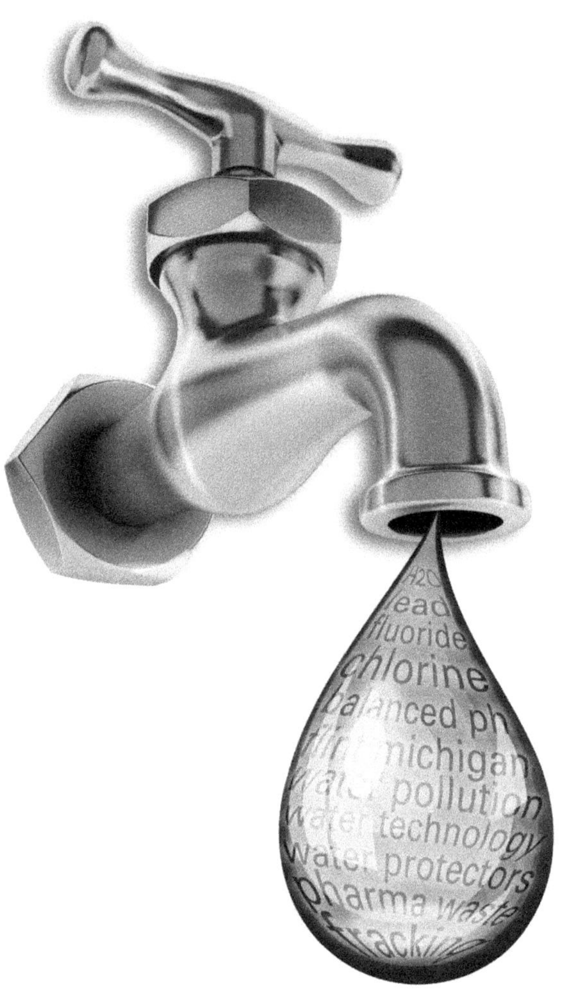

H2O
lead
fluoride
chlorine
balanced ph
flint michigan
water pollution
water technology
water protectors
pharma waste
fracking

CHAPTER 1

SOURCE OF THE PROBLEM

Source: As we take a look at the poor water quality issues that have hit major metro centers such as Flint, Michigan and Newark, New Jersey, we examine the source of these issues and what some are doing to protect the most important natural resource vital to the existence of the human race.

While the world's population grows and our available sources of clean drinkable freshwater dwindle, the critical demand to find ways to preserve and protect our current water supplies has rapidly increased. Alternatives to cleaning used and polluted water supplies are now being explored. Public Utility and technology companies are eager to develop the ability to filter recycled water for reuse as fresh water supplies continue to be maxed out.

According to the U.S. Geological Survey, only 2.5% of the all of Earth's water supply is fresh water. The main sources of available drinkable fresh water mainly come from glaciers, ice caps, ground ice and permafrost, as well as lakes and ground water. We, as a society, have not done enough to preserve and protect it. Ironically, we have continued to increase pollution of our rivers and lakes.

Only about half of the world's population has access to clean drinking water, leaving the other 3 billion people to fight for a source of quality water. According to United Nations Educational, Scientific and Cultural Organization (UNESCO) 783 million people have no access to *any* clean water sources and are left to rely on "dirty" water or no water at all.

Many believe this to be a problem that only plagues impoverished countries, those lacking infrastructure and societies with undeveloped economies. That stereo-typical outlook has been crushed by the recent developments which now haunt the cities of Flint, Michigan and Newark, New Jersey. One of the richest developed nations in the world also struggles to deliver quality fresh water to its citizens.

Flint discovered its dilemma in May 2014. It was only disclosed to a few circles in the political arena. Neighboring Detroit residents attended rallies where candidates for governor would be speaking. They were determined to share their concerns for the tainted water that was now coming out of their faucets.

Nearly a year later, the truth was finally revealed. Lead was contaminating the water. The culprit of this inescapable problem was the aged infrastructure. The city had switched the location of its water supply. However, it never added any anti-corrosive agents to the new water supply as was required. This misstep was the singular contributor which caused aging infrastructure to break down much faster than expected. The exposed lead from old lead pipes was carried to the point of distribution, the faucets in people's homes. Not only did Flint and Detroit face the challenge of 'finding' quality water free of chemicals, they had to create a method to 'deliver' this water to residents. This had to be accomplished without additional poison entering the water supply at the source of delivery or through its aging infrastructure.

The city faced a huge uphill battle in financing the replacement of its unfit pipes. Detroit and its neighboring suburbs have lost half of their population over the last twenty years. This means fewer residents are available to spread the cost of replacing pipes and infrastructure.

Flint is not alone. Newark, New Jersey has now joined the ranks of cities that are dealing with a contaminated water supply. It is no surprise that one of the largest metro areas in the Garden State is facing serious issues with their water supply. New Jersey is known as the state that has the most environmental issues. It has more superfund sites listed with the EPA than any other state.

New Jersey took measures to protect valuable clean drinking water supplies when its governing body passed the Highlands Water Protection and Planning Act, in 2004. This law was to slow urban sprawl and protect hundreds of thousands of acres that supply the majority of the state's residents with fresh drinking water. It included land surrounding some of the state's largest reservoirs, natural preserves, and wildlife sanctuaries. It protected these areas from over development.

In Newark, aging infrastructure was the culprit. However, there was a larger issue that no one dared to mention. There was a contributing factor that was more of a risk than aging infrastructure. In the foot hills of the highlands are reservoirs which collect runoff water from neighboring regions of West Milford, Ringwood, and Wanaque. At the center of years of environmental controversy was the former sight of Ford's dump, where paint and other related chemicals were discarded in the heart of the Ramapo Mountains.

Located just miles from this dump site is New Jersey's largest fresh water supply. It has taken years for the by-products and contaminates to reach this water supply. Some contaminates have been found as far away as Totowa, New Jersey. Deemed too costly to clean-up, both the New Jersey State Governor and the US EPA have shuffled this issue along, with little or no action to resolve this monumental crisis. Residents in this area continue to fight for environmental justice.

Tragically, it is deemed too little too late, as traces of these chemical compounds are now making their way to faucets around the state. This issue was originally covered in my former article, *"Is the Garden State Really Green?"*

With little public money available to solve these issues now and with the clock ticking, how do we solve the problems facing these two cities? It is estimated by Flint Michigan Mayor Karen Weaver, that it could cost as much as $1.5 billion dollars to correct the issues in Flint and Detroit suburbs.

Until the problem is solved at the source, New Jersey will also be left with a tainted water supply originating from the Ramapo Mountains for generations to come. It is paramount we find solutions to abate these dilemmas.

The World Green Energy Symposium 2016 was recently held in Washington, DC. During his address on Water Solutions, Paul R. Puckorius, CEO of Puckoriusof & Associates Inc., was asked how to deal with the Flint water situation. Puckorius answered:

"…One of the best ways to tackle the situation in Flint and now in Newark is invest into filtration at the source of water coming into the home and at point of delivery/usage. This will cost much less and allow for the cities to plan infrastructure upgrades and funding."

Currently, residents of Flint are receiving bottled water, which in reality is inadequate. The faucets and taps in Newark schools are turned off. However, a remedy is needed for the long term solution for these epic challenges. Stay tuned as we investigate other stories regarding water supply concerns in the United States and how we should begin to address this very important issue.

CHAPTER 2

DISTRIBUTION AND DELIVERY

Source: Water must sometimes travel over hundreds of miles to reach those who depend on it. What is the real price of distribution and delivery of fresh drinking water, and how do we protect clean drinking water from being contaminated during its journey to its final destination?

Water; without it our society comes to a screeching halt. This natural resource is necessary for our existence and our way of life depends upon it. From manufacturing to food production, water is a vital requirement for feeding our planet and build the modern conveniences of today. Water is the most precious resource on planet Earth. Yet we put our future at risk every time we either waste this valuable commodity or abuse it with pollutants.

Half of the United States depends on clean, fresh water sources that must be distributed from another area of the country. Sometimes it must travel hundreds of miles from its original source. During this journey, water faces the risk of contamination. Aging infrastructure is a major factor of lead contamination in water supplies in both Flint, Michigan and Newark, New Jersey.

A stressed economy, metro centers with aged infrastructure and a shrinking population compound the mounting complications of how to fund and fix decaying pipes and waterways. In Flint, it is not the distance which the water must travel that is the issue, but how the water must get to end users. Flint's Mayor, Karen Weaver, stated that it would take over $1.5 billion dollars to update the infrastructure that carries water to residents and businesses in the region.

In a report published on March 21, 2016, it was stated that the aging pipes that carried Flint's water supply to residents contained lead and were contaminating the water. The decaying pipes leaked traces of lead into the water supply, which would then affect the quality of water at the faucet. The complete report can be reviewed at:

http://www.michigan.gov/documents/snyder/FWATF_FINAL_REPORT_21March2016_517805_7.pdf

In other parts of the United States, such as the barren southwest, entire communities are facing major water shortages. This includes South West States of Arizona,

New Mexico, Colorado, and Utah. Each have faced rapid population growth in the cities of Las Vegas, Phoenix, Santa Fe, and Salt Lake City, which are major urban metro centers that rely on water sources as far away as Colorado.

As these urban center populations grow, infrastructure and the demand for clean fresh water increases. The main supply, the Colorado River, is over taxed and dwindled. New residents who relocate to these metro areas often bring with them plant life and urban landscape not native or natural to the area. As more homes and lawns are added to the system, the demand for water rises. Residents must make choices about curb appeal sacrifices in the name of water conservation.

Over the past few years, California has also faced an ongoing water crisis. The amount of record rainfall needed to naturally sustain southern California and its agriculture industry has been far below the norms. Urban zones like Los Angeles and San Diego have seen a rise in population growth. With the lack of rainfall, California is facing serious water shortages.

California produces 70% of the nation's fresh fruits and nuts, and 55% of the nation's vegetable supply. Many parts of the state have instituted water restrictions on watering lawns and washing cars and sidewalks. However, these practices are too little too late.

Presently California is getting water from water supplies that are tied to the Sierra Mountains of Nevada to meet growing water demands.

The further clean drinking water must travel, the greater its risk of becoming contaminated. In West Virginia, the Elk River was recently polluted by a manufacturing company dumping pollutants into the waterway. This water is the main source of drinking water for Central West Virginia. The further water must travel to the point of delivery, the more filtration systems are needed to deem it potable.

New York City, home to over 8.5 million people, gets its drinking water from Upstate New York. Water must travel up to 125 miles before it is processed, filtered and then sent to kitchens and bathrooms in the five boroughs. What standards are in place to assure that the water which has traveled hundreds of miles is the same or better quality as it is at the source?

In the case of New York City, since most of the water is naturally filtered through a series of watershed areas, the water is relatively clean. The city did begin to build a state-of-the-art water filtration plant known as the Croton Water Filtration Project. There are some aging issues within the infrastructure, resulting in over 36 million gallons of water lost to leakage each day.

In Flint, it is a much different story. In order to save money, Flint Michigan began to source its water from the Flint River, which contains significant amount of chlorides;

corrosive agents to lead pipes. The filtration systems in place were in fact functional but when the water had traveled through the aging infrastructure, lead was present in the tap water. Since this issue was brought to light, the city of Flint returned to its original water source, Lake Huron.

A variety of technological devices are currently being explored regarding purification and reprocessing of waste water into a usable water source. These devices would be applied to building cooling systems and refrigeration, irrigation for agriculture, and water for manufacturing or maintenance needs. The outcome would provide clean, fresh water for drinking that can be preserved solely for human consumption.

Gray water is water from showers, laundry, sinks, and other non-sewage sources. Although this water cannot be digested by humans, it can be reused for toilets, irrigation, laundry and car washes. Both biological and mechanical filtration systems are utilized in filtering and purifying gray water so it can be used again.

Sea and ocean water are being considered in places located near these sources where fresh water is scarce. The process of removing saline, salt, and other harmful agents from sea or salt water is already used on ships and submarines. One percent of the world's population relies on this energy-intensive process for clean drinking water. However, it is estimated by 2025, over 14% of the world's population will be getting their drinking water from desalination.

As our population grows and our access to clean drinking water dwindles, the price of bottled water will skyrocket. Our society has been trained by consumer habit and a strong marketing effort. We now expect to purchase a case of bottled water when shopping for groceries. Though these sources of water seem to be a bit better and more trusted than scooping up water from our local lake or stream, not all bottled water is created equal.

CHAPTER 3

QUANTITY VERSUS QUALITY

Source: With hundreds of bottled water brands available and a large spectrum of prices, how does one choose a brand of bottled water? We provide insight into what makes a quality bottled water worth its price and how to evaluate a good deal on bottled water.

Who would have thought people today would be paying as much as three dollars for a single bottle of water? Thirty years ago a person would simply put a glass under their faucet and drink what came out.

Our society took clean, fresh, drinking water completely for granted. Now because so many of our local fresh water sources have been polluted, much of the population has resorted to purchasing water from the supermarket.

How good is the water on sale for $2.99 for a case of 24; 16 ounce bottles, and why is some even more expensive? Is there a process for making the best purchasing decisions on the quality of water we choose to put in our bodies or is it purely economics that dictate our choice for consumption? With so many brands and selections, how does a consumer choose the right bottled water?

The bottled water industry is a $9 billion industry. Pepsi's Aquafina is the largest in the business, followed by Coke's Dasani, and Nestlé's Poland Spring coming in third. There are some valid questions worth considering when choosing the type of water to buy. Are you actually getting the best quality of water when you purchase a famous brand product? Is a good price a good choice?

First, you have to consider the source of the water. Where does it comes from? Most of the cost effective, or in some consumers' minds, "cheap" water, is nothing more than filtered and refined municipal water. This means the water comes from public sources. Companies pay to access this water.

There is much advertising that tries to convince consumers that these waters come from other sources. For instance, some of these waters may be labeled with packaging that shows ice caps or mountain springs or rivers. As you read the fine print, the truth is revealed that the water comes from municipal sources. Other wording such as "natural" and "purified" create the illusion that these waters are as high a quality as some of their competitors. To know exactly what you are getting, a consumer must know the difference in the types of waters that are available and the quality of their sources.

Some of the best water comes from springs. One type of spring is an Artesian well. This is water that comes from a contained isolated source from deep beneath layers of rock and sand. The water is above the actual water aquifer and is not influenced by any man made water sources such as municipal water wells. Bottled waters that fall into this category include H2O Energy Flow and Fiji water. This water is viewed as some of the best water a consumer can buy. Usually these sources are well protected and are miles away from any industrial, commercial, and residential zones.

Some springs are accessible to the public. If tested and known to be sources of clean water, they can be the places to secure the best drinking water. There are springs throughout the country, such as Headwaters Spring in Mount Shasta and Red Rock Spring north of San Francisco. People flock to fill 5-gallon jugs with water that is cleaner than most types of purified tap water.

Purified water is water that has passed through an extensive filtration process. Other names for water in this category are distilled water, deionized water, or purified drinking water. Most of these waters come from municipal water sources which are processed through large commercial filtration systems. These systems are usually comprised of both mechanical and chemical filtering processes. This is the lowest quality of bottled water a consumer can purchase.

Mineral water is water that contains minerals and trace elements from its natural source. No minerals or chemicals can be added to this water. All minerals must be disclosed and this water must be monitored on a regular basis. No more than 250 parts per million may be detected in this water before it must be purified.

"Drinking water," is just another way of marketing bottled water. This water must pass the sniff test for humans to be allowed to consume it. It may be used for other purposes such as cooking, bathing, or laundry. Sweeteners and chemicals are prohibited from being added to these waters. Sometimes flavors are added. However, the trace amounts of flavoring are minimal so they can remain bottled water and not marketed as a soda or juice.

Some waters have a balanced pH. This is a measurement calculating acid and alkaline conditions. The ideal condition for drinking water is a pH of 7.8. Trace minerals that are important for the body are calcium and magnesium. Waters that contain these trace minerals are usually considered higher end water.

Other indicators that a water source is pure and of high quality are that the label of the product will provide additional information including whether or not the water is arsenic free, chlorine free, BPA free, MTBE free, chromium 6 free, and trace pharmaceuticals free. These are items one could expect to be in water that comes from municipal sources.

With this information about the types and qualities of bottled water now provided, you can make an informed decision whether water is a cost or an investment. If price is the most important factor in your buying choices, then you will not be getting the top shelf, best quality water available.

When you look at the valuable commodity, water, as a cost, you are shutting out any product information about which water is actually better for your health. If you view buying habits as investments, you are probably willing to pay a little more for quality. As the consumer, ultimately the choice is yours. Know the type of water you are getting when you chose price over quality.

Other alternative water supplies which have grown in popularity over the past few years include the collection of rain water. Rain barrels have been set up to collect runoff water for garden irrigation, washing cars, and property maintenance.

Cisterns and cistern systems have also made a comeback. These types of systems consist of large tanks or sealed reservoir systems that collect water from rain, snow melts, runoff, and fountains. Water is then redirected into these storage tanks. Systems can be simple with no or minimal filtration when the water is for non-human consumption such as irrigation, washing of cars, or laundry. Some systems are significant in nature and outfitted with commercial filtration units so that the water can be used for drinking, cooking, and bathing.

Many homes in America have their own well water. A well is either dug or drilled until the drilling rig hits an aquifer or water source. A pump, usually powered by electricity, is then placed in the well. It pumps the water to the top of the well for distribution to the faucet. Homes located in rural areas usually have wells as water sources.

The only cost for this source is the maintenance and powering of the actual well equipment. However, if the water is considered hard water and contains heavy metals such as iron, a filtration system is added to purify the water to make it more palatable.

What price can you put on the most important natural resource known to man? Is there a price one is willing to pay to sacrifice clean fresh drinking water sources? We all have a responsibility to keep our lakes and rivers free of pollution and garbage. We need to be mindful not to damage or pollute ground water sources. Our very next glass of water depends on it.

CHAPTER 4-

SO...WHAT'S IN YOUR WATER?

Source: With all of the recent concerns about the water crisis in Flint Michigan and in Newark, New Jersey, one must wonder, "So, what's in my water?" In this chapter we will examine the chemicals usually found in municipal water supplies and the chemicals used to purify and filter water. This will provide a complete picture of the real threats that exist in our water supply.

People do not generally consider what is added to their water. It is the million-dollar question as it relates to chemicals commonly found in drinking water supplies. Many of these chemicals are introduced to water supplies by man to help purify the water. Some minerals and chemicals are natural to water supplies and depend on the region in which the well source is located. We will review each chemical, the purpose it serves, and the danger it poses.

Water fluoridation is a process in which controlled amounts of fluoride are added to municipal water supplies to reduce tooth decay. This practice began in the United States and spread to other countries. Although naturally found around the world in some water supplies, fluoride is now added to numerous water supplies in 25 other countries.

According to the World Health Organization, there are over a half a billion people who consume water that is floridated. Two hundred million of them are in the United States. The WHO advocates fluoridation of public water supplies and claims health benefits.

This practice has resulted in controversy. Since the 1940's, community activists have raised concerns about the true nature and safety of the fluoridation process. Dr. Paul Connett, who has come out against the practice, shared his professional views as to why the general public should oppose this practice and demand a change in policy. He claims that fluoride is classified as a drug by the Food and Drug Administration and adds no extra benefits to drinking water supplies.

It has been argued that ethical boundaries have been violated by adding a known drug to water supplies in the name of social good. This chemical has damaging consequences over time.

In his study released on September 2012, Dr. Paul Connett reveals the harmful effects of fluoride. He claims that fluoride is not an essential nutrient to the human body.

Fluoride can accumulate in the human body, especially in vital organs such as the kidneys. Dr. Connett believes that there are no health benefits to humans ingesting this chemical and that many young children are over exposed to fluoride. This chemical may be doing more harm than good by discoloring children's teeth.

The National Research Council has discovered that too much fluoride exposure over time will have a profound effect on the brain, damaging brain cells and function. The Environmental Protection Agency has listed fluoride among the top 100 chemicals in which there is "substantial evidence of developmental neurotoxicity."

Another familiar chemical often found in public water sources is chlorine. Chlorine is a corrosive, poisonous, greenish-yellow gas that has a suffocating odor and is two and a half times heavier than air. This toxic chemical is part of the group of elements known as halogens. When combined with metals, halogens become halides. When chlorine is processed and manufactured commercially, it produces free chlorine, hydrogen, and sodium hydroxide. This manufactured product is then compressed into a liquid and packaged. It is added to drinking water, fountains, swimming pools, and other water sources used by humans. The purpose is to control and destroy bacteria.

Chlorine exposure may increase the risk of getting cancer. The American Journal of Public Health has published a report conducted by medical researchers from the Medical

College of Wisconsin. This report revealed that people who drank tap water on a regular basis containing high levels of chlorine and chlorine by-products have a greater risk of developing bladder and rectal cancers than those individuals who do not use such water supplies. The study indicates that 8-10% of all bladder cancer cases and up to eighteen percent of rectal cancer cases are a result of long term consumption of these chemical agents.

Lead is at the center of controversies in both Flint Michigan's water supply crisis and the crisis in the city schools of Newark, New Jersey. In both cases, lead deposits and lead contamination were results of aging infrastructure. The water supply delivery systems leaked and bled lead from the aging water pipes.

Lead is a heavy metal that can cause blood and lead poisoning. Many young children have needed medical attention in both cities as a result of the lead exposure. Lead can also negatively affect the brain and nervous system.

Polychlorinated biphenyls were commonly used as a coolant for various types of equipment, reducing fluid for machine operations and is found in heart transfer liquids. By 1979 this chemical was banned in the United States and subsequently by other international regulatory bodies in 2001. Rivers are one of the most contaminated water sources affected by PCB's, which are highly toxic. The thyroid is one area of the body adversely affected by PCB's.

The EPA has linked PCB's found in contaminated soil and water to cancer. The Great Lakes, sources of drinking water, were found to have high concentrations of PCB's due to industrial manufacturing nearby. These factories had released the chemical which made it into the lake's sludge.

Chemical fertilizers are another major contributor to the challenge of managing clean drinking water. In nearly every lake community where residents manicure their property, of lawn fertilizers leaches their way into local water sources such as lakes, rivers, and streams. Natural run off causes the fertilizers to enter the water. Many of these common lawn fertilizers contain nitrogen, phosphates, magnesium, potassium, sulfur, and petrochemicals. These chemicals cause an increase in vegetation growth in lakes and streams, compromising the natural eco-system. When this happens, the presence of oxygen in the water is diminished and replaced by other chemical by-products.

Other common contaminates found in municipal and recycled water supplies are trace pharmaceuticals. How does prescription medicine end up in the water supply? Until a few years ago, a common practice was to dispose of unused or expired prescription medication down the toilet or garbage disposal. This medication would eventually dissolve in the waste water supply where it was treated and recycled for other uses.

A study conducted by the Associated Press revealed that drinking water for more than 41 million Americans was affected by high levels of trace pharmaceuticals found in the water supplies. Although filtration of water is required, there is little regulation that mandates the processes or systems to filter out trace pharmaceuticals. Currently, there is no federal law that requires public water to be tested, monitored, and/or treated for trace pharmaceuticals. Even some bottled water, which comes from municipal public water sources, has been found to contain drug contaminates.

In addition, there are pollutants and chemicals which are added to water supplies by natural processes and atmospheric circumstances. Air pollution and its contributors can make their way into clean lakes and streams in rain cloud molecules. Acid rain is created when carbon dioxide, sulfur dioxide, and nitrogen dioxide mix together to form a light acid. When rain water molecules mix with these acidic chemicals in the atmosphere, acid rain is created. The acid rain then falls to the ground and into oceans lakes and rivers.

It is important to know exactly what is in your water. If you get your tap water from a municipal public water source, you can obtain a yearly report from your local Municipal Utilities Authority. All test results of public water sources should be on file and available upon request. If you have your own private well, you can hire a company to conduct a primary and secondary well water quality test. These tests are only a few hundred dollars and can provide significant information about your own ground water source. This test in some states is now mandatory when selling or buying a home.

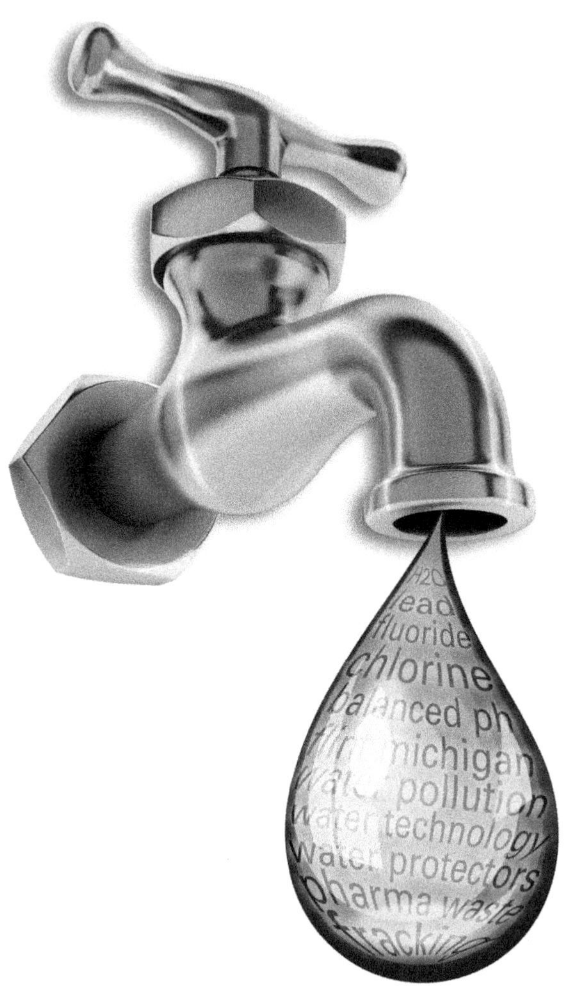

H2O
lead
fluoride
chlorine
balanced ph
flint michigan
water pollution
water technology
water protectors
pharma waste
fracking

CHAPTER 5

WHERE DOES THE BEST WATER COME FROM?

Source: So many bottled water companies claim that their water comes from the best sources. All of the different types of water available for human consumption can be confusing. We investigate to find where some of the best sources come from, spanning the world in search of the planet's freshest and cleanest water supplies.

Although 70% of the Earth's surface is covered with water, only 1% is available for fresh drinking water. Where does the best water come from? Words like "all natural" and "spring water" can seem very appealing. However, to find the best sources of unpolluted water, researchers have traveled to many parts of the world. To understand where the best sources of water originate, we need to dig a little deeper and sometimes we need to look at earth's highest peaks. Most sources of drinking water that come from the faucet originate from one of two places, surface water or ground water.

Surface water is water collected from lakes, reservoirs, rivers, and streams. Most major urban centers rely on these for their fresh drinking water. Ground water comes from aquifers consisting of highly permeable rocks, soil, and sand. Water can be extracted through wells that pump water to the surface or found as natural fed springs. In places where these resources have been over taxed, waste water is treated and put back into water distribution systems. In some areas where fresh water is scarce, salt water is refined into fresh water through the process of desalination.

Let us examine ground water a little more closely. Ground water is water that is located under the surface, locked up in spaces called pores, which are between rocks, sand, soil. They can also be located between cracks and crevices deep below the earth's surface. In some instances, these water supplies are under such immense pressure that they can spring up through the surface. In most cases, a well must be dug and water must be pumped to the surface.

Most of these water pockets are trapped inside aquifers. There are two common types of aquifers, sand and gravel aquifers, and bedrock aquifers. In the sand and gravel aquifer, water is trapped between the individual chunks of gravel and grains of sand. In bedrock aquifers, most water is found along fractures within the rock, joints, voids, and valleys between different slides of rock formations.

Bedrock aquifer water is the most difficult to release because it is surrounded by solid material. It is purer than sand and gravel aquifer water because the bedrock blocks harmful materials from seeping into these spaces.

Ground water is replenished through a natural cycle. Rain water, melting snow and ice seep through the layers of soil making their way into these natural aquifers. Most water that enters topsoil layers is absorbed by plant life. Some water is held by the soil, Topsoil acts as a natural sponge. The rest of the water moves down into the layers of the aquifer. In order for water to flow to a well or a stream, an aquifer must be at its maximum potential.

The surface of these aquifers, which leak water into wells, streams, and springs, is called the water table. This is the top of where water levels are located. In cases where there is an over-abundance of surface water, streams, ponds and lakes begin to develop.

This natural factory; an eco-system that regenerates water and produces our most valuable resource, is extremely sensitive. Our main concerns now become how to properly handle waste management, surface runoff, and limit the number of harmful toxins introduced into this cycle.

Surface water is usually categorized as water that comes from streams, rivers, lakes, and reservoirs. Surface water is preferred since it is less expensive to extract, collect, and distribute to households. Because surface water is more available and does not have any natural barriers to help filter pollution or containments, it must be properly treated using both chemical and mechanical filtration processes.

Surface water is more sensitive and susceptible to pollution. Brownsfields, which are properties contaminated by pollution, are monitored to prevent run off contamination from seeping into surface water supplies.

Artesian wells are another water source. Pipes carry underground water that is under natural pressure. This pressure pushes the water to the surface. Scientist say this type of well defies the laws of gravity because the pressure that builds up between layers of rock has a chance to subside when water finds a path to the surface.

Artesian well water is considered one of the purest waters because it is naturally filtered as it passes through porous rock. Artesian wells are very popular because no infrastructure is needed to access the water. These wells need minimal filtration and the water can be brought to the surface with little or no effort.

The purest water supply, which could provide two-thirds of the world's fresh drinking water for human consumption, is trapped inside frozen ice caps, icebergs, and glaciers. Countries within the Arctic and Antarctic Circles and countries with the highest elevations and the most snowfall have the most valuable water. Unfortunately, it takes many years for this water to become accessible.

The Institute of Earth Sciences, located at Germany's Heidelberg University, claims that the cleanest and purest water source within the Arctic Circle is located in the small village of Elmvale, Ontario. The reason is that this water is accessible and contains less atmospheric lead than any other source within the Arctic Circle.

Water located under Mt. Fuji in Japan is considered one of the purest sources in the Pacific. Located under the famous volcano, just 600 meters below the surface, is the natural spring that provides this fresh water.

The Andes Mountains and valleys contain some of the purest water in the world due to the minimal urban development. Being far from manufacturing and close to ice caps, snow caps, and glaciers, the water that makes it into these aquifers has had minimal human influence, such as waste, pollution, toxic run off, etc.

The countries of Canada, Finland, Switzerland, Fiji, Norway, Austria, Sweden, and New Zealand have the richest and purest water sources in the world. Both ground water and surface water are of the highest quality.

Countries with the worst water quality include Mexico, Indonesia, Tajikistan, Mongolia, and India. This is due to the high concentrations of manmade pollution that found its way into water sources. Years of abusive land management practices, over-use of fertilizers and chemicals, poor waste management, manufacturing and mining pollution have been major contributing factors compromising water supplies.

Poor water quality has a significant impact on health. Many poisonous and harmful bacteria and viruses thrive in dirty water conditions. Insects that carry harmful diseases find haven in polluted water sources. As human beings, we have a responsibility to diminish as much of our negative influences on fresh water sources as possible and curb practices that compromise both surface and ground water resources. To ignore the findings of professionals, advocates, and schools of thought about the importance of preserving fresh water sources will only lead to our own demise. We should not discount these warnings. We should take responsibility for protecting the most important natural resource.

CHAPTER 6

THE MOST ENDANGERED FRESH DRINKING WATER SOURCES IN THE WORLD

Source: Fresh, clean drinking water is the most sought after natural resource on the planet. With over seven billion people calling planet earth home and a limited supply of available, uncontaminated water sources, clean, fresh drinking water seems to be disappearing at an alarming rate. We will examine the most endangered drinking water sources on the planet and how this contamination affects the surrounding communities.

With a growing global population and dwindling resources, there is serious international concern that clean, fresh drinking water will no longer be available to sustain the needs in our modern world. Though planet earth's surface is covered by 70% water, only 2.5% of that surface is fresh water. Water is not a luxury, although for many, it may seem like it is.

Water is the very essence of what sustains life. As our population grows, the demand for fresh water increases. This puts a stress on current supplies. In some parts of the world, the well has dried up, while others face extinction.

There are five major regions in the world where ground water depletion is reaching critical levels. The five most threatened population centers of the world are Northwest India, Northeastern China, Northeastern Pakistan, California's Central Valley, and the United States Mid-west.

Not only is it important for these populated areas to have fresh, clean drinking water, these regions rely on clean water for the agriculture that sustains the region. Water sources in deep aquifers have been highly affected by over use and over drilling of wells. These areas have fossil aquifers. Fossil aquifers are not rechargeable. Rainwater or ground water from other sources cannot enter these aquifers. Once these aquifers are depleted, there will be no more water to pump to the surface.

Several lakes have become a statistic as a result of overuse of water and climate change. In China, Poyang Lake was one of the world's largest freshwater lakes located in the northern providence of Jiangxi, China.

Today it is nothing more than a marsh across which people can walk. The 1737 square mile lake fell victim to drainage as it was needed for drinking water. The lack of rainfall has made the restoration of this main water source even less hopeful.

Lake Mead is the largest man-made lake which is a result of the construction of the Hoover Dam. Lake Mead is located on the boarder of Nevada and Arizona. Due to drought and overuse, Lake Mead has been rapidly decreasing in size. It is the main source of clean, fresh drinking water for over 20 million people who live in Arizona, Nevada, and California. Snow fall from the Rocky Mountains, which sit tall in Colorado, Wyoming, and Utah, is the main source of water replenishing Lake Mead. However, Lake Mead has dropped 120 feet between 2000 and 2015.

The Aral Sea, which once shared boarders with Kazakhstan and Uzbekistan, is now a desert. During the mid-2000's, Russia diverted the sea to serve agriculture and irrigation projects. The rivers that once fed the Aral Sea were dammed or diverted as the demand for pure drinking water and water for agriculture continued to rise. This body of water not only provided drinking water but also supplied the region with a daily catch of fresh fish. With the disappearance of the Aral Sea, the fishing industry also vanished. The only sign left of what was once a vibrant waterway are old boats and vessels that litter the former lake bottom.

In Africa, a lake that was important to serve many is also endangered. Lake Chad has had a history of expansion and contraction depending on long dry seasons between rainfalls. Lake Chad has always been a main stay in providing fresh water to over 68 million people in over four countries. What makes this lake so unique is that it is shallow. Any change in its depth sounds off the alarm due to its unique feature that it is only about 35 feet at its deepest point. With so much of the lake's feeders diverted for clean drinking water or farming, Lake Chad's life expectancy is estimated to disappear by 2037.

Lakes are not the only waterways threatened by climate change, over draining for fresh drinking water, and pollution. Many rivers and important waterways for supplying millions of people with clean drinking water are affected as well.

The Colorado River is on the endangered list of bodies of water threatened by overuse and changing weather patterns. The Colorado River is fed by snow and ice that trickles down from the peaks of the snow-capped Rocky Mountains. Climate change has brought droughts to the region. Many communities rely on the Colorado River for their main source of clean, fresh drinking water.

The Colorado River water sources have also been diverted to serve larger population centers, including Las Vegas, Los Angeles, San Diego, and other metro areas of the Southwest. Many of the river's tributaries have been tapped for agricultural use, further stressing the river.

In Southwest Asia, the Indus River is carefully monitored as fresh water supplies dwindle each year. This river flows through Pakistan and India, and is the main source of unpolluted drinking water to a population of both countries. This river begins in the Tibetan Plateau and makes its way to the Indian Ocean. The Indus is a national treasure as it served as a main source of water for the ancient world.

Currently, the river sustains local fishing economies, farming, and manufacturing. During modern times, the river has been dammed in several spots, impeding travel from one end of the river to the other. Before environmental regulation, many manufacturing sites set up shop along the river and then discharged their waste into the flowing water. The demand on the Indus has caused the river to drain significantly. Some sections of the river no longer flow.

The Murry River in Australia is listed in critical condition. The Murry is vital to sustaining life. It is a main source of water to the diverse eco-system of plants, birds, fish and animals that live in the surrounding area. The Murry River is a main source of pure drinking water for most of the suburbs and metro area of Sydney and Melbourne. The Murry has been impacted by the stresses of modern society because of a growing population in these metro areas. The Australian government has begun to mitigate and restore parts of the river, limiting settlements in highly sensitive areas along this body of water.

Glaciers are the purest and freshest source of clean drinking water on earth. Fresh water is locked in chambers of frozen ice until warm weather allows melting snow to trickle down from the mountains into valleys, rivers, streams, and lakes. Climate change, the demand on more clean water sources, and pollution together have created the perfect storm for harming glaciers around the world.

The Alps play host to Europe's main source of fresh, clean drinking water. Located deep in the Alps is the famed Matterhorn Glacier. Since the 1960's the ice cap on this mountain has become so diminished that one can see the sharp distinction of rock formations instead of ice caps. Over two-thirds of the glacier and its surrounding sister glaciers have been lost. This region supplies over 40% of the clean water to Europe. These trends are primary concerns of the green movement in Europe.

Our very own Muir Glacier, located in Alaska, may soon be added to the extinction list of glaciers that are already disappearing from mountain tops around the world. The Muir feeds many rivers and streams vital to the Salmon industry. With lower runoff, some rivers may become dry stone beds. This is a disastrous trend that would affect the entire eco-system of Alaska. The Muir was never a flowing body of water. It was a frozen chunk of water stuck in time. Entering the post-modern era, the Muir is now more of a body of water than a polar ice cap.

In parts of the Andes Mountains, glaciers and ice caps have been disappearing at an alarming rate. The Chacaltaya glacier completely disappeared in 2015. Its neighboring glaciers are facing the same fate. The ski resorts that once covered this region are now ghost towns. The more serious matter beyond recreation is supplying pure, consumable drinking water to the region, and their continued ability to feed rivers and streams used to supply hydro-electric power for neighboring metro areas.

Whether you believe in global warming, climate change, or the influence man has on the planet, one thing is for certain, without clean, fresh water sources, life on Earth, as we know it, will not exist. Water is the essence of life. Without it, crops cannot grow, livestock cannot be supported, there would be no mass manufacturing of goods and life would cease to exist.

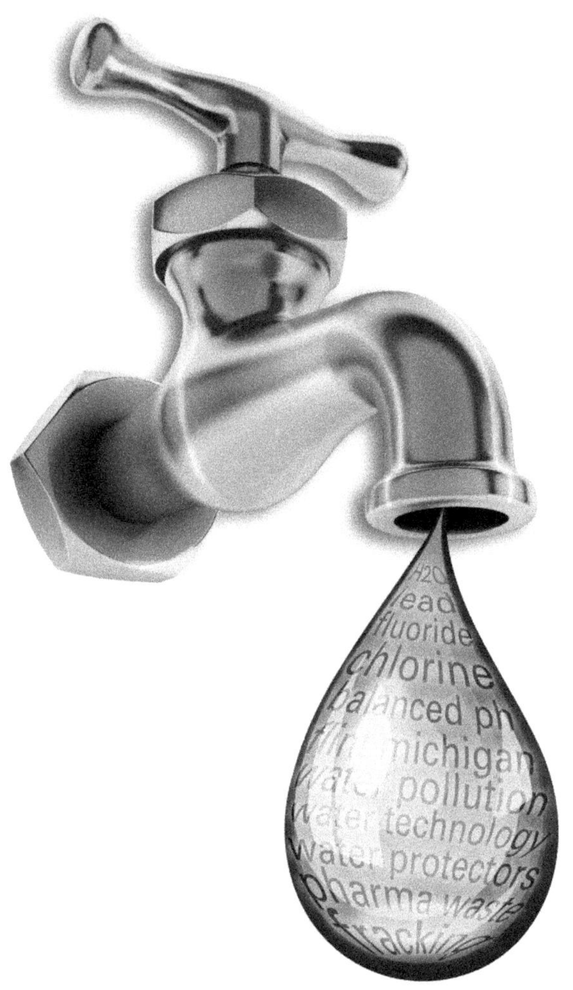

H2O
lead
fluoride
chlorine
balanced ph
michigan
water pollution
water technology
water protectors
pharma waste
fracking

CHAPTER 7

THE REAL PRICE FOR QUALITY DRINKING WATER

Source: The true cost of quality drinking water varies depending on the source of the water, its destination, who controls and supplies the water, and the varied ways water is consumed.

There are other costs that we as a society must consider as part of the price of water. These costs may not be reflected on a balance sheet. Here we will take a look at some of the long term costs as well as the real price we pay for clean drinking water.

Consumers consider the cost of water to be whatever the price is at the store, or the price of public sources delivered to the home. Those costs are just the tip of the iceberg. Some costs move beyond the balance sheet and typical accounting measures.

If we add up what an individual will pay per liter or gallon, and we add that number to all of the indirect factors not on a financial spreadsheet, the cost and price we pay for clean drinking water is much higher.

Over the past decade, major corporations have begun to distribute water for profit, resulting in a significant increase in the cost. There are two models which are utilized in the distribution of public-municipal water. The first model is when the people own the water supply. The local water supply is controlled and maintained by a local municipal water authority, usually comprised of a committee of either elected or appointed officials.

This model is a true municipal public utility. Prices per gallon delivered to households are mandated to be capped so that the regulatory body does not make a profit. The price per gallon varies depending on the geographic location of the municipality. For example, the Borough of Sparta, New Jersey charges residents $4.50 per 1000 gallons for this service.

The second public water source is when a local or regional municipality or government contracts water to be supplied to residents through a major corporation. This model has come with controversy. Most people believe that having access to quality, fresh drinking water is a human right. They are against companies profiting from supplying this basic human need.

Companies like Suez and United States Water are private corporations that make contracts to supply local municipalities with water. These companies are responsible to ensure the water they are delivering meets or exceeds regulatory guidelines. Consumers need assurance that better water quality for less money will occur. In some cases, residents saw a major increase in their monthly water bills when corporations controlled the water supply.

For example, cities contracted with United Water saw a price increase of over $1 more per 1000 gallons compared to the price of water supplied by the municipality. United Water's average rate is $5.50 per 1000 gallons.

A private well is deemed the most cost effective way for a homeowner to obtain a clean fresh water source. The use of wells has been abandoned in preference to public water in most post-modern day era suburban communities. There are still large pockets of suburban communities and vast tracks of rural settlements maintaining private wells providing the property owner a guaranteed source of quality fresh water.

The cost of a well varies by how deep a well must be drilled before the drill bit taps into the underground water table or aquifer. In the northeast, installation of a well could range from $15 to $30 per foot for a well that is 100 to 400 feet below the surface. There are the additional costs of the well pump, piping, and maintenance. These costs range from $2500 to $10,000. Typically, a well pump life span is 15 years and can cost an average $700 to replace.

If you have either municipal water or your own well, you will likely need a filtration system to capture any undesired elements in your water supply. If your municipal public water source has aged infrastructure, or if your private well water is hard and full of iron or other mineral content, you will want to have a water softener system and filter system installed. The cost of these systems range from hundreds of dollars to thousands of dollars, depending on the degree of mitigation you need in order to resolve these issues.

According to Sundale Research, 66% of people in the United States purchase the majority of their drinking water either from a home delivery service or from the grocery store. The average five-gallon container will retail for $8 each. Households will also spend money on ready-to-go single use bottled water containers which vary in cost depending on size and quality. Most average brands of water sell a 24 pack of 16/20 ounce bottles for $4.99. If you purchase a structured water or specialty water, you can expect to pay up to that price per bottle. It depends on your personal preference and the quality of water you select. Considering the profits to be made in the water distribution industry, many companies push to be first in line to provide water to millions of people.

The agriculture industry often depends on irrigation from water sources for growing food. The same water supply meant for homes and local communities may be tapped for agriculture as well, even during times of drought and dry seasons. Some manufacturing facilities depend on water for processing products including metal, plastic, paper, clothing, as well as food products. Eventually the stresses of these demands put pressures on Mother Nature beyond the available supply of water. When this happens, and local water sources are depleted, officials must resort to sourcing water from distant locations. The cost of additional infrastructure and delivery will likely go to the consumer. This is the case in California where water shortages have become the norm and freshwater must be imported from neighboring states. Much of the Southwest depends on water which originates from the Colorado River. In an area that has experienced a rise in temperatures and decline in rain fall, the Colorado River is already at its limit. Diverting more water from the river to suburbs of California comes with a premium price per gallon to consumers.

Pollution also costs us in the long run. The cost of clean-up of an oil or chemical spill is an open checkbook. There is no way to truly know the price to clean pollutants that make their way into water supplies, lakes, rivers and streams. These costs are astronomical. Pollution has drastic effects on eco-systems and influences other localized cottage industries that make their living depending on the land around them. Fishing and gaming are affected when oil spills and other pollutants are distributed into these sensitive habitats, limiting the supply of clean food.

Agriculture is also affected because polluted water is unhealthy for growing local crops. The soil that surrounds these contaminated waterways becomes tainted and unable to sustain life. What price can you put on a track of land or what once was a clean freshwater supply which no longer can be used because of man's own irresponsibility in handling waste not meant for nature?

Polluted water comes with a heavy price tag to our personal health. The World Health Organization estimates that polluted water sources affects 1.8 billion people each year. It is responsible for the majority of diseases in undeveloped and developing countries. Illnesses such as dysentery, diarrhea, and cholera are costly and can have deadly consequences when not addressed. Five hundred thousand deaths are related to diseases and illnesses that originate from polluted water. In these regions of the world, sources of drinking water and sewage are passed along in the same waterway.

There is an ancient Indian proverb which says,

"We do not inherit the earth from our ancestors; we are borrowing it from our children."

This reflects the attitude and the approach we should consider in lessening our environmental impact on water supplies. We are putting future generations at risk from the consequences of our actions and our lack of resolutions to these challenges. The cost is drastic when we do not soberly consider water preservation and conservation. There is no price tag that can be assigned to the moral responsibility we have to assure that our children and our children's children enjoy the basic human right to clean, fresh drinking water.

CHAPTER 8

YOU ARE WHAT YOU DRINK

Source: The human body is made up of 60-70% water. The amount and the quality of water a person consumes directly correlates to the quality of their health. Because water is necessary for life, it is imperative that we request and accept only the best quality of fresh drinking water for our consumption. Water enters the body in a variety of ways. These include drinking, food we consume and the water in which we bathe. We will take a closer look at why we must be diligent in clean water consumption and how it influences the human body.

There is an old saying, "You are what you eat." This includes the liquids an individual consumes.

According to the Mayo Clinic, the human body is made up of 60% to 70% water. A person should be very conscientious in choosing the quality of the water which he or she consumes. The amount of water a person needs depends on age, health, activity level, and physical location.

Studies show that an adult should consume between six and eight glasses of water a day. These studies vary due to a number of factors, including the focus group's age, fitness, and physical location. If you live in warmer climates where the human body perspires more, you will need to drink more water than someone in a colder climate. Thirteen cups of water are recommended for men and nine cups are recommended for women per day.

Water is essential for life. It is a natural filter that helps our body flush out unwanted toxins. Water carries nutrients and minerals to our cells and is responsible for keeping the nose, throat, and ears moist.

Whenever we sweat, breath, urinate or make a bowl movement, water leaves our body. This water needs to be replenished. Dehydration occurs when a person loses large quantities of water. This may be caused by exercise, the environment, illness other health conditions, pregnancy, breastfeeding or lack of food.

Acting as the "oil" and the "glue" of our body, water helps us in many ways. It protects our organs and tissues. Water helps flush unwanted toxins from our organs, especially our digestive system. It carries toxins from our liver and kidneys, lessening their harmful effects.

When our digestive system has sufficient water, the processes of breaking down and utilizing food and disposing of unwanted waste occurs efficently. Adequate water consumption helps prevent constipation.

Our joints rely on fluid to minimize wear. Water serves as the lubricant for them to work properly. Water helps regulate our internal temperature. Our normal body temperature is 98.6 degrees Fahrenheit. Water acts much like antifreeze, a coolant to our body. A warm drink can warm the body. Water helps cool the body from fever, over exertion and high environmental temperatures. The body's systems depend on water to function properly.

Water carries oxygen to the body's cells. This is why some experts believe structured water is the best water to consume. Dr. Gerald Pollack from the University Washington, conducted a number of studies on water, including a search to gain a better understanding of how water affects the body. In an interview with fellow colleague, Dr. Joseph Mercola, in January 2011, Dr. Pollack made a profound announcement that structured water is best for the human body.

Dr. Pollack's research reveals the importance of having water that is structured and balanced with an ideal pH, due to the form and functionality of water itself, including how it works within the human body. One of water's main functions is to carry oxygen to the body's cells. Water should have a balanced pH, such as H2O Energy Flow, the less acidic and the more alkaline water is, the better it is for you. Alkaline water will carry more oxygen than acidic water, thus the more balanced pH the better.

Not all health professionals, nutritionists, and scientists agree that structured water is the healthiest. However, Dr. Pollack has kept skeptics on their toes. His research and studies have revealed a number of facts now disclosed formally. Dr. Pollack shares:

"In other words, there was a particular absorption of energy at a particular wavelength that's absolutely characteristic of the structured water," and, "That makes me think that there is a good possibility that the water really has the capability of retaining that structure over a long time... Therefore, it's possible that if you drink water that has this structure, it might be good for your health."

Dr. Pollack also says, *"I know there is a lot of skepticism about that, but from a physical point of view, it's entirely possible."*

Dr. Pollack has studied water for several decades and has written a number of books on the subject. He and his team are currently exploring the effects of frequency imprinting, how it affects the quality and molecular structure of water, and its impact on the body.

Why choose water instead of other drinks? Drinks such as soda, contain a number of chemicals and sugars that are known to wreak havoc on the human body, especially if consumed in large quantities. Studies have shown that excessive consumption of soda may result in weight gain, diabetes, and other digestive issues. Soda contains many acids that do more harm than good and soda should be consumed in moderation.

Alcohol is another toxic beverage that can be harmful to the body. It has a volatile effect on the body's organs. Excessive alcohol use can lead to cancers of the mouth, throat, esophagus and liver. In addition, it may damage vital organs.

Sports drinks such as Gatorade and PowerAde are not replacements for water themselves. These sugary sports beverages contain high levels of electrolytes and sodium. These may provide temporary relief from dehydration. However, they should be offset with the recommended water consumption when over-exerting the body during physical work, fitness, or participation in sports. Many energy drinks also contain caffeine for a temporary boost.

Coffee and tea drinkers are encouraged to drink more water because caffeine dehydrates the body by stimulating the kidneys to eliminate fluid. It is not the coffee that directly dehydrates. It is the caffeine that causes the diuretic effect resulting in the production of more urine. For this reason the consumption of soda, sports drinks, and other highly caffeinated drinks should be limited.

There is no replacement or substitute for water. You should be aware and monitor the amounts of water you consume and the quality of the water you choose to drink. Since your body needs water to function properly, it is so important to ensure the water you are drinking comes from a viable proven source. If the water at your tap is not the quality you desire for maximized health, consider other options. A water filter or a new water source may be the answer.

CHAPTER 9

THE IMPORTANCE OF A PH BALANCED WATER

Source: Since such a high percentage of your body is water, your pH level is an important indicator of your general health. Before you purchase your next bottle of water, understand the importance of purchasing bottled water that has a balanced pH level. What does that mean to you? Why is that so important? We examine the answers to these questions below.

To aid in selecting water based on its pH level, there must be an understanding of what pH means. The pH value is an indicator of water's acidity or alkalinity. When testing pure water that has not been processed, the water should have a pH value of seven. Water with a lower pH rating is acidic, and a pH higher than seven would indicate the water is alkaline. Clean, fresh, surface water has a range of pH values from 6.5 to 8.5.

Water with a lower pH level than seven is acidic and is corrosive to pipes, plumbing, and the human body. Acidic water may contain metal ions including; iron, copper, magnesium, lead, zinc, and other heavy metals. Other toxic elements carried in water are mercury, cadmium, and petro-based substances. Heavy metals are toxic to the human body when exposure to them occurs on a regular basis.

According to Dr. Edward Group of the Global Healing Center, the human body actually needs a small trace of metals. However, our bodies, through exposure to unclean water, food, and air, take in far more heavy metals than what is healthy. Too much exposure to heavy metals will lead to heavy metal poisoning. The body's cellular levels experience stress due to these foreign contaminates.

Dr. Group's list of heavy metals to avoid are usually carried into the body by drinking water. This water has a low pH level and may include aluminum, mercury and lead. Additionally, Dr. Group lists in his journal a number of foods and products that also contain these toxic elements.

Acidic water is easily recognized by its bitter taste. Where pH levels are extremely low, the water has a metallic taste. This may indicate that the pH levels in the water are so low that the water must be exposed to an extensive filtration process. This process may include both a mechanical-physical filtration and a chemical filtration. Chemical filtration may include the use of salt, chlorine, and other bio-agents.

Water that is alkaline may contain important minerals that the human body needs, such as magnesium or calcium. Water located deep in the earth, in the ground water table or in artesian wells will likely contain these minerals dissolved from the rocks resulting in acidic water. In some cases, water bottling manufacturers will ionize the water to make it more alkaline. Even if there are minerals present, the process of ionizing the water will lower the pH level.

Alkaline water can be divided into two categories; naturally alkaline and artificially alkaline. Alkaline water that is natural is infused with minerals through a natural process in which the minerals enter the water at the source. Like ground water or water from an artesian well, these water sources that are deep in the rocks or ground contain minerals that have leached into the water. Artificial alkaline water has been ionized by a mechanical/chemical process. This process can be very costly if the natural pH of the water is too low and acidic.

Flowing water creates the highest concentration of natural alkaline water. In its natural setting, water flows over rocks in streams and rivers, picking up minerals contained in these rocks. No man made mechanical processes are involved.

Artesian wells, which are protected by rock formations deep in the earth, also experience a natural mixing process of minerals when rain water seeps in and filters through the rocks into these deep cavern wells. The pH value of alkaline water is an indicator of its ability to neutralize acid.

Too much alkalinity in water can be counterproductive. Alkaline water that is infused with high concentration of minerals can cause excessive drying of the skin. Some minerals will remove oils from the skin. If your household water is too alkaline, you may choose to incorporate a water filtration or water softener system. These can neutralize the mineral content of the water. Using lime can soften the water and neutralize some of the minerals in water. In some cases, salt is used as a chemical filter to lessen the concentration of minerals that make water's pH too high.

When purchasing bottled water, it is important to note the pH level of the brand you have chosen. Some companies do not specify the pH of their water. You can research if pH testing has been conducted on their water. If you are seriously concerned about the pH level of the water in popular brands sold at the grocery store, you can purchase one bottle of each brand. Then using a home pH level water testing kit, you can determine the pH of each brand.

Water brands such as H2O Energy Flow and Fiji Water, clearly state their pH levels on their bottles. H2O Energy Flow claims that their water has a pH level of 7.8. Fiji brand states that the Fiji brand water has a pH value of 7.7. There have been many independent tests conducted on major brands of bottled water. The results of these tests can be found online.

Taking an inventory of food consumed and noting its total pH; can help a person decide what water would be their healthiest choice. There are a host of programs and metric calculations online that will provide further information on this subject.

There are many debates between health and medical professionals versus the bottle water industry regarding what is the best water and why. I encourage each person to do their own research about what water will be best for them. When making a purchasing decision, it boils down to an individual's personal choice.

A water filter or purification system are alternative choices to consuming bottled water. These systems are mentioned later on in this book.

Knowing the human body is made up of 60% to 70% water, and knowing how much water your body needs based on your age, health, activities, fitness, and diet, aside from your medical professionals, you are the authority in knowing what type of water will best work for you.

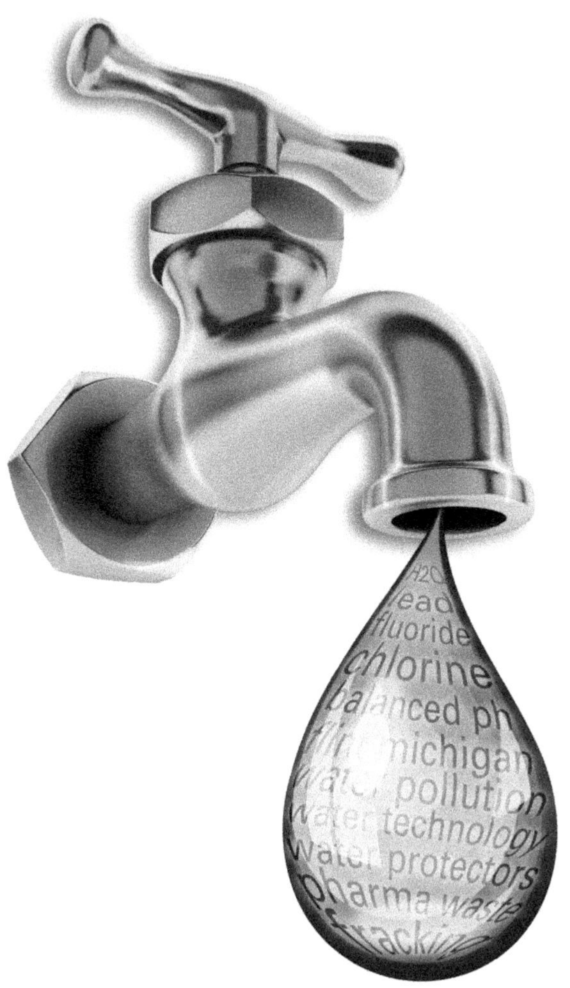

H2O
lead
fluoride
chlorine
balanced ph
flint michigan
water pollution
water technology
water protectors
pharma waste
fracking

CHAPTER 10

PUTTING WATER TO WORK FOR YOU

Source: We put water to work for us constantly. Whether we are adding soap to clean our bodies, our homes, or adding detergent to clean clothing, water's chemical makeup is responsible for its ability to clean. In this chapter we will explore how water works with specific chemical agents we use in daily activities.

Water is one of our most valuable resources and without it life cannot exist. It is also one of the most powerful resources available to mankind. Unfortunately, this natural resource is often taken for granted, as we tend to overlook its significance in our busy day to day lives. It is important for us to have a clear understanding of how water works on our behalf. Then we can gauge and temper our use to better conserve and preserve this precious resource. Understanding the science may help. Water is a sensitive compound easily influenced by chemicals added to it or its environment. To get a greater understanding of this concept, we must review water's basic elements.

Water is a compound made up of two elements. It consists of two hydrogen atoms and one oxygen atom. Its chemical formula is H2O. Hydrogen is the lightest and most prevalent element in the universe. It is colorless, tasteless, odorless, non-toxic and non-metallic. It is extremely combustible and a highly reactive, unstable element.

Oxygen, is the third most plentiful element. It too is highly reactive. It is necessary for human life and for our respiratory system to function. When hydrogen combines with oxygen, it forms a water molecule.

Knowing the components of water, and how each individual element works, we can now understand the bigger picture of how water can be influenced by outside factors.

When detergent or soap is added to water, it changes the structure of the water molecules and how they react. The general assumption is that the soap or detergent is what cleans our clothing and linens. That is not the case. It is the water that cleans our clothing and linens.

Water is at its most powerful state when it is broken down into small molecule chains and clusters. This allows it to penetrate even the minutest of crevasses in the surface of an object. Water must be fractured to achieve this function and cannot fracture itself. Water must be fractured so that its molecules and clusters can be reduced into small enough parts to seep into the pores of the surfaces. When the water molecules reach into these pores, the dirt or soil attaches and blends with the water. The water carries away the dirt. Soap and detergent are added to the water to fracture it into parts. Some detergent and soaps are more effective than others.

The purpose of cleaning agents such as potassium hydroxide, sodium hydroxide, potassium carbonate, and surfactants, when applied and mixed with water, is to disrupt the water molecules. The large clusters of the water molecules are broken into parts. This allows the water molecules to become small enough to penetrate the surface which is being cleaned. Contrary to belief, this is actually how ones clothing and or other household surfaces become clean.

There are two basic foundational agents used in most soaps and cleaners to fracture water. Potassium chloride (KCI) is a well-known agent in most soaps. It has the ability to react with water and force water to fracture its molecules into a ionized state. Potassium chloride, also referred to as a lye solution, is the main ingredient in lye soap. Potassium on a molecular level has a great impact on a water molecule. It is the volatility of mixing these two materials together that factures water into its parts allowing it to be an effective cleaner. Potassium chloride is the most common cleaning agent because less water is needed to clean effectively.

The other common base of most soaps and cleaners is sodium hydroxide (NaOH). Sodium hydroxide is also known as caustic soda and lye. This cleaning agent has been used to balance the pH level of water. A higher pH level in water results in less damage to water infrastructure pipes and plumbing. It minimizes the amount of harmful metals that can contaminate water supplies used for human consumption. Sodium hydroxide is a powerful cleaning agents. Too much sodium hydroxide can result in unpalatable drinking water.

Cleaning products that are derived from surfactants can be effective cleaners while also friendly to the environment. Many surfactants, including plant based surfactants, are non-toxic and biodegradable. For this reason, cleaners that are surfactant based are the safest and most eco-friendly. This cleaning mixture can usually be disposed of down the drain with little or no harmful effect to drinking water supplies.

Potassium can be useful when it is combined in another form with water and safe to consume. This is known as potassium carbonate (K2CO3). Most sports drinks, such as Gatorade and PowerAde, contain this electrolyte. When water is infused with potassium carbonate, a reaction occurs. When consumed, the body absorbs the liquid molecules faster, allowing for a more rapid hydration of the cells of the body to occur.

Water mixed with natural elements can also be a great agent for cleaning surfaces due to the chemical reaction which occurs between water and the introduced agent.

Some home remedies for cleaning products include mixing distilled white vinegar with water to wipe down surfaces and floors. For glass, water with lemon juice has had its advocacy by individuals looking to steer away from chemicals in the home.

Water's awesome power is also released when the surface tension of water is reduced to the point where each water molecule is broken into its monatomic state. The result is harnessing the individual molecules as energy sources.

HHO is a term that means hydrogen + hydrogen + oxygen. It is a fuel source to power an engine originally designed for petro fuels (gas or diesel). A more refined version of hydrogen fuel from water sources is H2, where the oxygen molecule has been targeted and eliminated. For years, inventors and scientists have researched and developed systems and technologies aimed at capturing the water molecule as a fuel source to power vehicles.

Some of the most well-known scholars in the field include the legendary Stanley Meyer, Yull Brown (Brown's Gas), and Jerry Smith, who patented their ideas on this very subject matter.

When put under pressure, water has many other applications. It is used in a pressure washer. Water is forced through a small nozzle under immense pressure washing away a filthy, caked on surface covered in dirt and grease. Water, when boiled and put under pressure, creates a pressurized steam that can power equipment, vehicles, and even trains, as they did at in the early 20th century.

Using water as a tool for our needs is a result of harnessing its energy when disrupted, influenced, or combined with an outside source. Water's energy is most effective when it goes from a chemical change to a mechanical change.

Becoming better educated concerning how water, when mixed with various cleaning agents, not only benefits us in our daily lives, but effects the environment as well, is the responsibility of everyone. With this information, we are reminded that what we mix in water to perform domestic and commercial tasks, will eventually end up back in the ground, possibly affecting the water sources themselves. This clearly supports the recommendation that people use agents that will have the least negative effect on the environment.

CHAPTER 11

WATER'S OTHER VALUABLE ROLES IN OUR MODERN SOCIETY

Source: To survive and thrive as a civilization, our reliance upon pure, uncontaminated water goes beyond our drinking needs. Society is also dependent upon clean water that comes from trusted sources for commercial-industrial consumption. So how much water is actually required to sustain our society's needs?

Too often our natural resources are taken for granted. Life today is so modernized and fast paced, that rarely do we take time to think about all of the ways we depend on water.

Whether this vital resource is for drinking, agriculture or for manufacturing products, water is a critical component of the operations of society. The lack of water in some countries is a matter of national security if they depend on neighboring nations. Many industries rely on water to manufacture its goods.

Water is essential for food production. Even sewage treatment is dependent on water to assist with our waste water management. So how much water is needed to sustain all the moving parts of our society? We will take a look at five essentials we need in order to maintain life.

Food production is vitally dependent on clean, fresh water supplies. In the United States alone, there are as much as 442 million acres of land dedicated to farming. These include growing food for humans and for livestock. Many of these crops rely on irrigation when rain falls short of delivering enough water throughout the growing season. Water for farming and gardening comes from many of the same sources, as our drinking water.

Agriculture and horticulture account for 80% of all ground water usage in many of the nation's regions, and up to 90% in some of the western states. In states such as California, Texas, Idaho, and Florida, agriculture is the largest consumer of water. Farm water usage is almost always freshwater. This results in a major stress on drinking water supplies. Water for agriculture eventually works its way back into the eco-system.

A substantial amount of energy is required to cool the production of thermoelectric energy, which is our second largest source of water consumption. This process of producing energy from thermoelectric involves the use of great amounts of water. Water is utilized to cool equipment that produces electric power. Heat exchangers circulate the water and then return it to its source.

Another form of water, steam, is used to turn turbine generators, resulting in the production of electric power. Not all of this water is fresh water. Some of it is salt water.

Water can also be used for hydro-electric power generation. Water for hydro-electric power comes by way of damming rivers and building hydro-electric power plants that are integrated into the falls of the river. A well-known example is the plant at the Niagara Falls. This was the first hydro-electric power plant in the United States. Niagara Falls relies on overflow from Lake Erie into the Niagara River as well as into Lake Ontario.

Another example of water being put to work to generate electric power is the Hoover Dam. This dam is situated on the Colorado River between Nevada and Arizona. The Colorado River is fed water from melting glacier and ice caps located high in the Colorado Rockies.

Water is necessary for the manufacturing of many consumer goods, vehicles, and nearly all items we purchase as modern conveniences. Water is required for mixing paint, which may be used when painting building interiors.

Water is used to rinse away left over materials from manufacturing products, unwanted debris, and shavings or millings left behind by the manufacturing process. Water is also needed to supply these manufacturing facilities with fresh drinking water for employees, showers in locker rooms and restroom toilet facilities.

Many manufacturing sites have air conditioning units to ensure a temperature controlled environment. Water is used as part of the air conditioning-cooling process. These facilities may use water for heating as well.

When manufacturing raw goods such as metals or plastic, water is one of the most important components of the process. Water is used to cool steel to strengthen it. Hot steel is dipped in water immediately after the metal has been formed, thus tempering it.

Utilized as a cleaning agent, water is sometimes applied under high pressure to prep materials for their next phase of manufacturing. It may be mixed with a chemical to sterilize metal for food or medical use.

Water is an ingredient used to make plastic and to clean plastic parts. Its heavy use in the process of manufacturing on CNC machines is critical. Water is projected onto the surface of the widget being manufactured to cool the drill or laser cutter.

Water is in high demand in the construction industry. The manufacturing and application of cement and concrete rely upon it. Water is part of the process in making lumber and building materials. The construction industry depends on partners of mining and quarry for aggregate materials (stone, sand, rock) which are used in erecting buildings and manufacturing construction materials. Water is necessary for washing or filtering dust and impurities from aggregate materials.

Once buildings are constructed, approved and occupied, copious amounts of water is needed for maintenance, including irrigating of plants and grounds. Water use for landscaping must be uncontaminated. Golf courses are one of the largest consumers of fresh water for their buildings and grounds preservation.

One very controversial use of water pertains to the oil industry. This process is known as hydraulic fracturing, hydro-fracking, or fracking. A deep well is drilled far below the earth's surface into pockets where oil and gas preserves may be located. These pockets are found in very hard to reach places hidden inside either rock formations or softer material caught between large fissures of rock. Fracking fluid, usually consisting of water, other chemical agents, and sand, are put under high pressure then pumped into these crevices where oil and gas exist. This forces these substances to float to the surface.

Unfortunately, clean water is used to make the chemical mixture for fracking. There has been little effort to remediate the spent water resulting from this process. To make matters worse, this mixture, which includes toxic chemicals, is left in the ground. It seeps into ground water supplies, including private wells for drinking water.

Sewage treatment requires not only spent water, as it is part of the sewage, but fresh water that is added to help filter out contaminates. Sewage treatment in the United States is some of the most advanced in the world but it still requires a fresh water supply.

In some countries which do not have sophisticated and modern infrastructure, sewage is directly dumped into streams, rivers, lakes, harbors, and even water ways reserved for travel. As sewage is introduced into water sources reserved for drinking, larger problems arise. Unsanitary and poisoned water leads to health hazards, some of them catastrophic to entire populations.

Countries without adequate sources of unpolluted drinking water often lack the most fundamental base of an economic engine, manufacturing. Nations that lack water for manufacturing are at the mercy of trade agreements that determine how much their population will pay for goods and services from other nations.

Many countries in the Middle East have negligible water sources. They must develop marketable products to meet their economic needs. Some examples are tourism, information, technology, and fossil fuels, where fossil fuel exists. Many of these countries hope to be central distribution and entry points to the region for goods and services from Europe, China, and the US, to the Middle East.

There are far more uses of clean water than one often considers. As a society, we usually focus on what is in front of us, that which pours out of the faucet or comes out of the shower head. The hidden danger is that we waste water in many other areas of our lives.

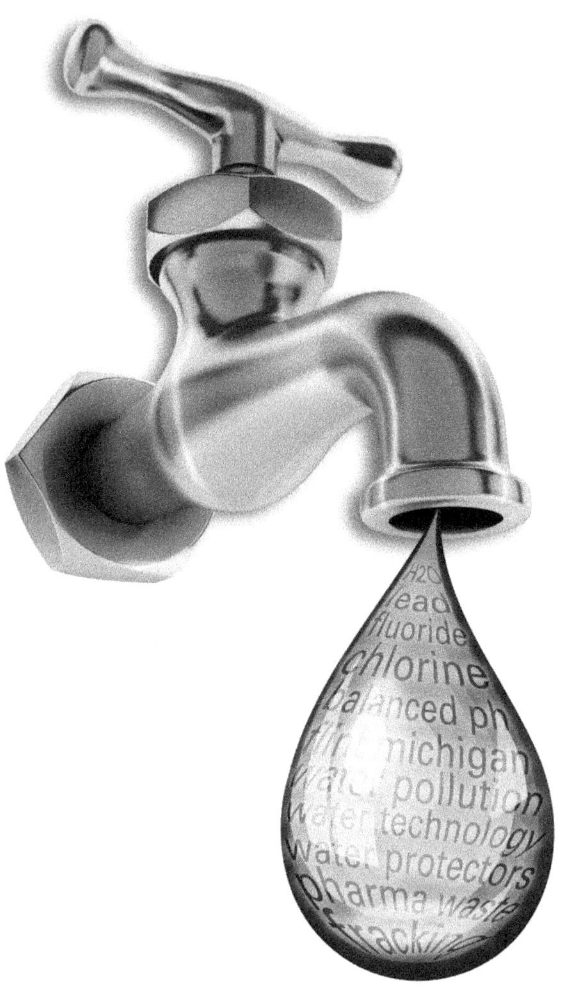

H2O
lead
fluoride
chlorine
balanced ph
michigan
water pollution
water technology
water protectors
pharma waste
fracking

CHAPTER 12

NEW TECHNOLOGY AIMED AT REDUCING WATER USAGE

Source: In order to preserve water, we must explore new ways to protect current water supplies. New technology may be the answer.

There have been many technological advances aimed at conserving water usage. They range from small home products to technology and systems for industrial use. All are focused on reducing our use of water.

Technology that helps us to live cleaner more convenient lives is constantly being developed. Areas of concentrated focus where technological advances and improvements are moving at a rapid pace are conservation, distribution, and treatment. Some areas of the world with the greatest needs have population spiraling out of control, placing new demands on available water supplies.

Some of these technologies are simple upgrades to already available water treatment devices in the home. Others, however, are completely innovative and radical by traditional standards. They are designed to handle water treatment and water conservation on a massive scale. Water conservation is nothing new. Methods and technologies have improved over time. New ideas have been instituted to use gray water when the situation does not require fresh water.

In the home, water is wasted most frequently in the bathroom. The toilet's design has not changed significantly. In some cases, the design of the internal parts of the tank have advanced. These toilets are more efficient as they take less water to operate. Tap and flush technology involves new regulators and float systems that allow more precise measurement of water used by the toilet. This is more advanced than the traditional float style regulator.

Another innovative, inexpensive technology is a toilet tank bag. It is simple to use and install. The bag is filled with water and placed in the tank of the toilet. The toilet bag displaces some of the water in the tank and allows the toilet to use less water with each flush.

The shower ranks second place in inefficient water use. Many faucet manufactures offer high efficiency faucet aerators, shower heads, and faucets. The purpose of these new faucets is to push the water around through powerful jets, providing a similar effect as if there is more water. These new faucet designs limit usage to ten gallons every ten minutes of shower time. That may not mean much to a household of one but would in a household of four or more. It is estimated that using these devices, a household of four to six people can save up to 400 gallons a month. That is over 4800 gallons of water a year.

Water flow valves are not standard in most homes. Home owners are largely unaware that they can regulate water usage by turning the knob of the valves. Closing the valve by 50% will result in savings. There are do-it-yourself water conservation kits. They range in price, with many under a few hundred dollars. These kits provide additional information on how to save on your monthly water usage and include a water flow meter that can measure consumption. Then a person can fine tune faucets, water valves, and appliances himself.

One of the latest at-home technologies is the installation of Smart Metering of water usage and the integration of Smart Watering controls. Regulating and measuring water usage has gone digital. These may save thousands of gallons of water per household per month. These meters are precise in measuring usage and control distribution.

Advancements in ultrasonic metering have led to many water utilities installing these new meters. Ultrasonic water metering and water controlling devices have no or minimal moving parts. This results in accurate usage data and less maintenance of the actual metering unit.

In commercial and industrial applications, the reuse of treated gray water has been gradually accepted. Gray water is often used to operate air conditioning and cooling units for buildings and businesses. The reuse of gray water has increased over the years. Gray water that has been filtered has been used for cooling systems, irrigation for farming and gardening, and at car washes.

More research has been conducted on how to extract soap and cleaners from gray water. In the future gray water may be recycled for use in other applications such as laundry. Gray water that has been treated is now being sold as a secondary water commodity by waste water treatment facilities and water utilities to help offset treatment cost. This is helping to conserve water for drinking, showers, and cooking.

Systems for collecting rain water have also grown in popularity. Before we understood the importance of rain water in our water system, we were unaware of the many opportunities to collect rain water. Parking lots with pervious surfaces, either by way of drainage or by using stone and brick instead of asphalt or concrete paving, have allowed commercial building owners to collect runoff rain water into giant holding tanks and cisterns. The collected water is then pumped to distribution locations. This water is recycled for irrigation of gardens and lawns or decorative fountains. Rain water has also been used for washing buildings and sidewalks.

Commercial businesses are encouraged to install ultra-low flow toilets and faucets to reduce water usage. Commercial buildings that use water to cool equipment can recycle gray water or switch to air cooled equipment for heating, air conditioning, and refrigeration. These types of buildings which still use steam boilers for heat, can upgrade the boiler to a machine that will use treated gray water. Many businesses have switched from fossil fuel and water driven utilities to electric to save on the use of water and energy.

New commercial dishwashers and ice machines use far less water than previously designed equipment. Although it may seem an expensive investment at first, use of the new equipment will save a restaurant, hotel, hospital, or school thousands of gallons of water a year. Commercial appliances with the EPA Water Sense decal have been tested and rated for water conservation and cost savings.

On the side of sustainable manufacturing are the many practices of water conservation mandated by law. Gone are the days when manufacturing sites were allowed to discharge waste water into local lakes, rivers, and streams. The old mindset was, "out of sight, out of mind," and polluted water was sent down the river and ended up as some else's environmental hazard.

Many manufacturing factories that exist today are responsible for proper hazardous waste disposal, separating waste from the water that carries it. Clean water is necessary in manufacturing goods and products such as plastics, vehicles, appliances, and other modern conveniences. Factories now filter and recycle water to be reused in processing raw goods.

Water treatment systems for recycling and reusing water have evolved over time. One of the most popular of today's latest systems is the Membrane Bioreactor system (MBR). It separates and treats different types of liquids and solids. Dissolved air floatation is a type of device that bubbles any contaminate to the surface of water. Then the frothy foam can be skimmed from the top surface of the water. Filtration and softening systems are most commonly found in factories.

These factories have oversized units that resemble those in homes. New systems known as reject recovery reverse osmosis water treatment systems, are being used in the soda and beverage industry. Sequencing batch recovery systems are found at engine and automobile manufacturing sites.

Water conservation now practiced by soil and water reclaiming conservation specialists include the replacement of protected wetlands and the reclaiming of these natural eco-systems. Research has found that wetlands have served us as a natural filter and barrier. The natural ecosystem of plants, animal life, and soil when mixed with water, naturally filters sediment and other materials carried downstream.

The wetlands function as a natural water purification system as they collect pollutants and heavy metals, well before these materials enter the natural waterways or ground water aquifers. Wetlands trap many of these harmful agents and either convert them to less harmful materials, or trap them and bury them in under-muck layers.

Surrounding ecosystems, where ground water has been restored, have aided in lessening the need for humanly created irrigation systems for lawns, gardens, and natural plant life found either at a well, decorated office complex or housing unit.

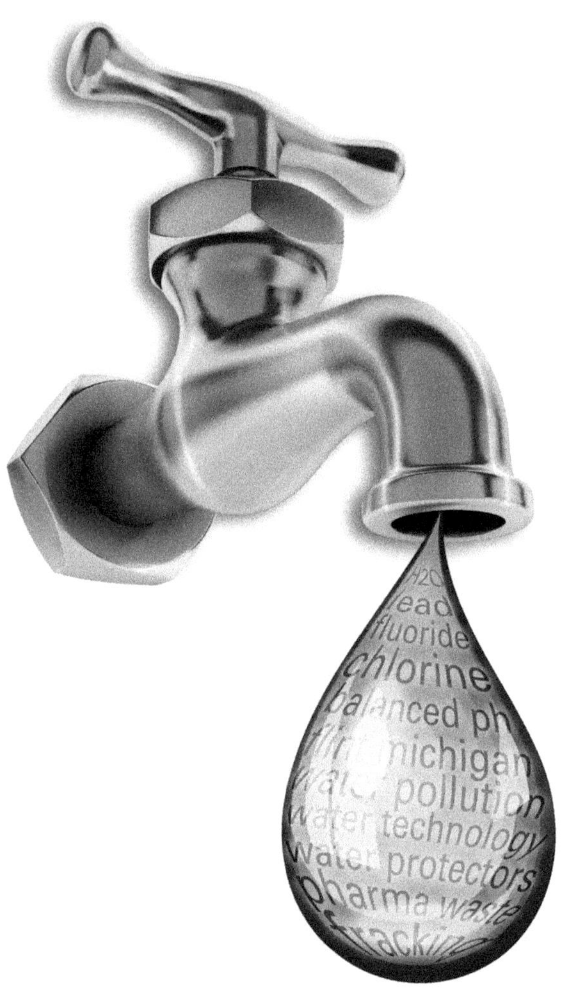
H2O
lead
fluoride
chlorine
balanced ph
flint michigan
water pollution
water technology
water protectors
pharma waste
fracking

CHAPTER 13

BATTLES ON THE WATERFRONT; WHERE ENVIRONMENT, INDUSTRY, AND PUBLIC POLICY CLASH

Source: It is not an easy task to balance the progress of industry and serve the public interest. Regulations, checks, and balances are needed to protect our natural lands and waterways. Public policy that shapes today's environmental justice sets the pace for how future environmental concerns will be handled. Some decisions come with unpopular consequences. We review some of the most recent and contentious battles in protecting our most important natural resource, water. Our society is very complex. There are over seven billion people on the planet. It is a fine balance between people, profits, and the planet. Our most important natural resource, clean, fresh drinking water, has come under siege in parts of the world where people are standing up for the planet over profits of industry. Government, which stands in the middle, has to choose the path of policy and must consider both sides of the equation.

On one side of the argument is industry which says that government is standing in the way of free enterprise. On the other side are the people who must live with the consequences of how industry affects the quality of our air, land, and water.

What happens when oil and water don't mix? It is a recipe for a very heated public policy debate, fueled by media frenzy and protest in the streets. There are a number of actions that have led to public outcry. Some of these battles are still ongoing without resolve in sight.

Fracking has become a hot topic. It pits public policy against large oil and gas companies which hope to capitalize on their investment in technology. This technique is a viable way to mine oil and gas from deep underground, hard to extract places such as shale, sandstone, and lime stone.

The economic boom resulting from fracking has ironically had an adverse effect on local communities, with neighbor fighting against neighbor. There are individuals who wish to cash in on their unearthed treasure fighting against those who understand and value the importance of preservation of water.

As you drive through New York's Sullivan County, beyond the stretch of road known as Hawk's Nest, there are visual reminders that the argument is alive and well. Signs that read "No Fracking" inside a circle with a strike through it are visible along driveways and on private properties which line Route 97, a major thoroughfare that runs along the Delaware River, outside Port Jervis, New York.

In opposition are the outpost and sight of testing rigs, survey teams, and oil and gas pipeline workers ready to make hay even when the sun is not shining. This is also a common sight in Bainbridge, New York, in the county of Chenango. It is a town located along the Susquehanna River. Both regions are at the center of debate for they contain two very valuable natural resources, natural gas energy deposits and fresh, clean drinking water.

In 2013, NJ Governor Chris Christie vetoed legislation that would ban processing and disposal of left over fracking material in New Jersey. Environmental activists gathered in protest before the statehouse to voice their displeasure for the Governor's action not to further protect New Jersey from the toxic material. This created a major outcry from environmental advocacy groups. New Jersey has become the state that holds the record for having the most environmental superfund sites in the nation.

Opponents of fracking note that there are no current technologies which are presently available to refine the waste product that separates the chemicals from the fresh water base used as a part of the fracking process.

Larry Ragonese, spokesman for the New Jersey Department of Environmental Protection would later share the following:

"There in fact might be minute areas where under the Utica shale may contain significant deposits of natural gas. These deposits are to known to be found mainly under the land in Upper Passaic County, Sussex County and Warren County; counties which rely on agriculture tourism for the majority of their local seasonal revenue."

These are also counties that constitute much of the basin that makes up the fresh water supply being managed by the Newark Watershed Conservation and Development Corporation. It is responsible for managing and delivering fresh drinking water to selected metro areas of the State.

On a national stage, land owners who wish to preserve the natural beauty and natural resources that either lie under their property or under neighboring properties, have utilized every method available to deter others from the practice. From lawsuits, temporary injunctions and restraining orders to large protests and acts of civil disobedience, opponents to fracking have made their voice well known.

David Pringle, Campaign Director for the Clean Water Action, New Jersey Chapter, (formally the New Jersey Environmental Federation), has been on the forefront of this National debate. He states:

"Fracking is not a bridge to the future, it's a direction off the cliff. Most people think that fracking is a cleaner alternative than coal, when in fact studies show otherwise."

In North Dakota near the South Dakota border, there is an even more heated contest between the people and industry. Both sides are asking the government to step in. The project known as the Dakota Access Pipeline (DAPL) has come under much criticism and has catapulted into the forefront of some media outlets covering the series of events.

Thousands of people have gathered to protest the construction of the new pipeline and have established an encampment since spring of 2016. Standing Rock Sioux Reservation plays host to ground zero of this matter.

The Standing Rock Sioux Tribe, the native people of this area, argue that the construction of the pipeline will disrupt their only source of clean, fresh drinking water because the pipeline is planned to be routed under the Missouri River.

The reservation's people rely on the Missouri for fishing, growing crops, and drinking water. The native population also advocates that other neighboring tribes and reservations will be affected if the project is allowed to continue. Members of the Standing Rock Sioux Tribe have stated that construction will disrupt the current natural environment and have catastrophic effects on ancient lands once used for hunting, fishing, and desecrate ancient burial sites.

The Natives are not alone. In neighboring states such as Iowa, farmers have filed into court seeking to deter the pipeline from entering their property. These people believe that once they have allowed the pipeline easement, there would be no limit to the government's and industries' continual land grab for more of the farmers' fields.

Not all people and groups hold the same concerns as the Sioux. The Texas based company, Energy Transfer Partners (ETP), is the lead party building the pipeline. ETP claims they have invested over 3.8 billion dollars into efforts to ship light, sweet, crude from fracking sites to refineries and other points of distribution. The company claims the pipeline is a good idea since it will reduce the amount of oil that is transported by rail or truck, subsequently reducing the amount of spills caused by transportation accidents.

While pipelines are designed to prevent leakage, leaks in this country increase with expanding capacity and aging infrastructure. In 2016 there were a number of leaks resulting in the spill of more than 250,000 gallons of crude oil or gasoline. An example is the Colonial Pipeline leak in Shelby County, Alabama. One of the large spills was from a Sunoco pipeline near Sweetwater, Texas that *was only one year old.*

The DAPL pipeline begins at the Bakken Oil Fields and will end in Illinois.

Energy Transfer Partners acquired all of the needed local, state, and federal permits to begin the project. In addition, it was given permission to enter private land not under the jurisdiction of the Standing Rock Sioux Reservation. In response, peaceful protests have continued. The original number of hundreds of native peoples swelled to thousands as environmentalists, military veterans, community activists, and members from other tribal nations joined to aid in the battle against the company.

One of the most ancient waterways in the world is still fought over today. The Tigris-Euphrates River system is considered the birth place of modern man. For over 5,000 years it has been a source of conflict. The Tigris and Euphrates span from eastern Turkey to Syria, Iraq, and the remaining Persian Gulf States.

The Taurus Mountains feed these two rivers with clean, fresh drinking water to the entire region. The first recorded water war was almost 4500 years ago. A dispute broke out between the ancient city-states of Lagash and Umma. These river systems have seen a number of horrific attacks on their waterways, including the Gulf conflicts of today.

These waterways have been stressed by the violent bombardment of cutting off fresh water to opposing parties. Also, with the decrease in rain fall and increase in rising populations, the Tigris and Euphrates Rivers have been tapped to the max, causing them to drain down.

According to the United Nations Environmental Program, over 90% of the original marshes of the two waterways have disappeared. These marshes acted as natural filters for these rivers. They dried up and have been destroyed as a result of over farming. Along with the marshes, a number of wildlife species have also disappeared.

Satellite images from 2003 to 2009 show that over one hundred million acres of clean fresh water have disappeared. Local groups and regional governments continue to spar over who has the rights to control these waterways. Each group attempts to dam up parts of the river system for their own use. Environmentalist groups have expressed their concern about damming up parts of these waterways. However, it is the locals that command the fate of these rivers. The issue that makes this battle for the Tigris and Euphrates unique is that there are so many groups fighting for this water spanning several countries.

As you can see, the fight over clean, fresh drinking water is nothing new. What is new are the types of additional threats these waterways face. We have a choice. We can continue to engage in conflict, or we can cooperate in finding a reasonable resolutions to these issues. Whatever the outcome, it will have a long lasting effect on future generations.

CHAPTER 14

NEW PUBLIC POLICIES AT WORK IN PROTECTING DRINKING WATER SOURCES

Source: As the demand rises for clean fresh drinking water and population centers continue to grow, legislative efforts to assure fresh water become a priority. The balance between the needs of the people and the needs of industry requires government to take a sharp look at these public interest debates and provide policy that protects this important resource. We will take a look at some of the latest policies that have been signed into law.

Aside from Federal law, many states have taken it upon themselves to institute new policies aimed at protecting clean water sources for farming and water.

Minnesota, "The Land of 10,000 Lakes," has proposed a new bill that focuses on protecting lakes and rivers. It is determined to clean up polluted waterways. The bill, known as the Stream Buffer Clarification Bill, revisited previous restrictions and clarified specific terms related to the treatment of development near streams. In general, the bill addresses the requirement for buffers of public drainage ditches only.

More specifically, it proposes the enforcement of purposeful pollution into storm drains and reviews alternative water quality practices that prevent overland flow to a water source. The Minnesota legislative body has continued to push for bonding for clean water projects. These would fund much needed infrastructure upgrades to avoid the colossal tragedy that plagues Flint, Michigan.

California led the country in signing new legislation to improve water quality and preserve water from over usage. The State Senate signed into law a bill that allows soil quality to be improved. The Healthy Soils Program reconditions soil so that less water is needed to sustain important crops.

California also sought to consolidate smaller public water authorities and private water plants with larger facilities and agencies. These entities did not have all of the financial resources to manage high standards in water quality. Merging smaller entities with larger water utilities will allow for these smaller facilities to upgrade equipment and systems.

Other measures to deter water abuse include a set of bills introduced by the California State Legistrature to enforce mandatory bands during drought or states of emergency. The state also adopted policies to improve and use storm water. Water usage data and cost can be monitored should water need to be diverted to another region.

The Sunshine State took time to examine comprehensive water policy in order to improve Florida's water quality standards. From these efforts came the Florida Springs and Aquifer Protection Act. Major previsions of this act include new standards for measuring springs and aquifers. If these minimal ground water flow rates or surface water levels are not met, then pumping from these sources must be halted until minimum limits are restored. This policy was designed so that groundwater would not be depleted to the point of a cataclysmic ecological disaster to surrounding eco-systems. The Florida Department of Environmental Regulation should begin to set new standards in place that address these issues.

Vermont has always been a leader in environmental protection. Vermont has put on its books new upgraded standards related to water quality and water management. New rules in water quality announced by the Vermont Department of Environmental Conservation include new policies on discharged water treatment standards for fresh water designated for drinking and pollution mitigation practices. The updates address enforcement actions for violators of rules.

The United States Congress has pushed for the Water Sources Development Act. It authorizes the Army Corp of Engineers to assist non-public entities conduct feasibility studies addressing future mitigation of privately managed waterways, funding of new projects, flood prevention, environmental mitigation, clean-up efforts and improvements to infrastructure.

How are foreign countries addressing these challenges? What policies have taken shape to assure the people of the world access to clean, fresh drinking water? Conferences and conventions that highlight water quality are plentiful but actual actions are slow.

The World Bank adopted a new policy that includes funding for clean water projects in parts of the world that lack this vital resource. It is known as Environmental and Social Framework. This plan was written to protect poor people who usually lack the ability to sustain clean water sources. Local groups are educated in practices to keep their new resources working. It lends money to groups responsible for maintaining these new facilities and utilities that provide water to the world's poor.

Some critics accuse the World Bank of capitalizing on this basic necessity of life which people need to survive. The program calls for monetizing new wells as a way to repay the funds borrowed for new uncontaminated water resource development. Critics claim that the policy is counterproductive because the very poor would be unable to pay. Putting water on a paying basis would only give false hope and shatter the dreams of communities incapable of paying for water.

To counter the World Bank, many Christian-based non-profit organizations have formed working groups or ministries that specialize in educating the poor on the importance of clean water practices and proper waste water management. They oversee the new construction of fresh water wells and filtration stations. Many of these groups are volunteers so the majority of the proceeds donated go directly to the effort of improving the quality of life. Some areas served by these ministries are in Africa, India, and South America.

Non-profit Christian groups such as The Water Project, have set up programs where donations and funds raised privately through grants go directly to sponsoring a new fresh water well drilled in Africa. These new wells are outfitted with filters and systems so that local villages and communities have access to pure water for drinking, bathing, and farming. This organization is not a religious organization but is run by Christians in the hope of improving the lives of people in the region by providing tools to take care of their own communities.

Governments under the banner of the European Union push for advancements in climate change policies. Global warming is believed to be the ultimate threat to precious uncontaminated water sources. Europe has upped their regulations on toxic vehicle emissions while also raising the bar for fuel economy standards. Fossil fuels contribute to the global warming effect.

Europe has always been ahead of the world in environmental policy and green technology by twenty plus years. Unlike policies in the Unites States which address enforcement of the laws, Europe takes a proactive approach to environmental justice. Europe sets standards, then they assist in funding solutions designed to help reduce the harmful effects of pollution. Europe has always been a leader in green technology and promotes green technology integration whenever possible.

Cities in countries where the central government has been criticized for acting too slowly have begun to institute policies as examples for other metro centers to follow. Some cities such as Paris, have banned vehicles within the city powered by diesel fuel by 2025. Paris was joined by Mexico City.

Members of the C40 Cities Climate Leadership Group are a network of people from the world's largest mega cities committed to addressing climate change. The group examines the cause and effect of environmental practices that need consideration for lessening society's impact on the planet. New initiatives and policies are developed.

Paris and Mexico City sit on the steering committee of the organization. Just three of the major metro cities from the Unites States are honored as "Innovator Cities."; Portland, Houston, and New Orleans. Boston and Los Angles are members of this C40. Europe leads the C40 Cities Climate Leadership Group with the most member cities, 20, followed by Asia.

Cities such as Amman, Jordan's National Capital City, which is also a member of C40, has had to cope and innovate due to the overwhelming number of refugees from neighboring countries still at war. With an explosion in population, the challenge of managing both clean and waste water becomes significant.

The group holds three conferences a year. Ecocity World Summit is the headline event. C4O is a resource tool for growing population centers to handle areas of operation within their city boundaries. These include business, economy, and innovation, as well as city intelligence, measurement, planning, and finance. Cities are encouraged to invest in major upgrades surrounding water works projects since some of these cities' infrastructures date back thousands of years.

Other proposed policies in recent water management practices have been directed towards privatizing water utilities. This is a profit driven model to drive down cost of operations and maintenance, while holding private operators to higher standards of delivering quality water. Regions of the world such as South America; have experienced heavy protest from the people. As a result, some countries have taken back some of their water utility operations.

History has proven, as long as humans are fighting for the God given right to clean, drinking water and the sources from which it comes, there will always be challenges and debate.

CHAPTER 15

METHODS FOR TESTING THE QUALITY OF WATER AT HOME

Source: Can you measure the quality of water that comes out of your faucet? If you have public water, the quality of the water is monitored, and by law, a report must be made available to the public.

What if you have your own well? What monitoring is in place to assure your own well is providing quality fresh drinking water? In some circumstances where your well or source of drinking water is located near a petro hydro-fracking site or landfill, there arise additional concerns related to the quality of the source of drinking water. Here we share a few methods on how you can test the quality of your water.

Water sustains our existence and is necessary for agriculture, manufacturing and most needs of modern society. We are generally unaware of all the areas in which water affects our lives, except when we are drinking, preparing a meal, or using water for hygiene.

Often we do not question the quality of the water that is delivered until we notice a visible difference in either the color, taste or odor. It is only then that we take action in addressing water quality concerns.

There are several methods an individual can use to test the quality of water coming from the tap. Some methods are complicated, costly yet are required by law when selling a home. Other methods are simple, with tests that can be conducted by a landlord, renter or homeowner. Regardless of one's budget, it is important to explore regular testing and monitor your own source of drinking water.

There are a number of do-it-yourself water quality test kits available at your local hardware store, home supply outlet, and online. They cost from a few dollars to hundreds of dollars, depending on the amount of factors the water test kit will review. In choosing a type of water quality test kit, it is vital to know what elements you will be testing. The most comprehensive do-it-yourself water quality test kits will check for heavy metals such as lead and iron, bacteria, harmful organisms, fertilizers, pollutants, and the water's pH level.

Many of these test kits use a grading system of color strip indicators that identify the levels of each factor. If a test kit has only one test strip, it is likely only testing the water's pH level. The best water quality kits enable you to test for multiple types of bacteria and pollutants. As you expose the test kit to the water from the tap, the color strips will change according to the mineral and bacteria content, as well as the host of pollutants that may be present.

Each test kit is unique. Some use a scale of color-coordinated coded keys for you to match the test bars against so you may have a better understanding to what is in your water source.

There are specific odors that will indicate additional important information. If the water has a heavy scent of bleach, it will have a high concentration of chlorine. The odor and concentration of chlorine usually disappears as the faucet runs. However, you may purchase a filter which aides in dissolving the chlorine content from the water.

If there is an odor of rotten eggs, it may indicate a serious problem. This odor indicates either a bacteria or sulfur pollutant in your water. To discover if the odor is an isolated issue such as a clogged pipe is a sign of something more, you must turn each faucet in the home on and off, checking each water outlet. If the smell continues throughout the entire home, you have a serious issue. The water source has been compromised before it has reached your home. If this is the case, contact your municipality water authority immediately.

If the water has a musty or earthy odor, it may indicate a clogged water drain and will need to be corrected.

A visual inspection of water may provide valuable information about the quality of your water. Pour water from the faucet into a clear glass container and hold it to a bright light. The light will reflect the contents of the water. If dark particles are present, it is a sign of decaying infrastructure, including metal and clay pipes that may need to be replaced or serviced.

Cloudy water is a sign of either too much calcium or magnesium. If the water has a green tint, it is most likely an algae build-up in pipes and waterways. Extreme amounts of sediment, such as grits and sand, may indicate that the water table or well has been compromised or is running dry. If your water is foamy, it may contain soap and detergents. Foam will rise to the top of the water sample and have a unique texture to the touch. Some water may have bubbles. However, these bubbles should disappear when the water sample has been stabilized.

New and unique methods of testing water quality have advanced over the last few years. You can take a small water sample in a glass jar and light a match to it. If the water puts the match out, the water is normal. If the surface of the water begins to take flame and burn, the water has been compromised by a petro spill or seepage of an underground oil tank. It is not recommend performing a flame test on your own. Leave this one to the professionals. UV light is also used to determine water quality. It is used at central water treatment plants to zap bacteria.

A black lamp may be used to search for specific minerals in a water sample. Pour the water sample in a dish. In the dark, wave the black lamp over the sample. If you notice florescent lights, your water will have a high concentration of zinc and other similar minerals.

Water should be tested and the results documented over time. This requires sterile glass jars with lids. Water samples are taken, tested, and stored. It is important to place a label on each sample with the date and time the water sample was taken and tested. Copies of results of each test should be kept on file. Should there be ongoing issues, it may be necessary to monitor water quality trends that will indicate what measures need to be taken to improve the quality of water.

A professional laboratory may oversee the testing and provide a report of their findings. In New Jersey, as well as many other states, there is a law called the Private Well Testing Act. It mandates testing a private well whenever a property changes ownership or is leased to a new tenant. This assures the next occupant that the water is safe for human consumption. If the quality of the water does not meet testing standards, the seller or landlord is responsible for remedying the situation. Replacing old plumbing and piping may resolve the problem. In some cases, a new well needs to be drilled. Testing can cost a thousand dollars and take up to two weeks. This is the most comprehensive test a property owner can perform and is a worth-while investment.

If you rely upon a public water source and desire to know the results of regular testing, contact your local municipal utilities authority. They are required to provide test results to the public. You can also obtain a Water Quality Report from the actual water provider. Many of these public water sources are under the command of a quasi-government agency or private corporation. A Water Quality Report is very extensive and lists all the requirements for which a public water provider is responsible. This information can be reviewed by accessing the US EPA website link at:

https://www.epa.gov/dwreginfo/drinking-water-regulatory-information

If water has a high concentration of bacteria, pollutants, heavy metals, or other types of contaminates, you may want to contact a professional to mitigate the issue as soon as possible. Most common water problems can be resolved by adding a series of filters and upgrading rusting and degrading plumbing infrastructure. The longer these issues persist, the costlier the remedy will be. If your local public water source is not measuring up to the quality within regulatory standards, you may demand the agency or public water utility to address the problem at once.

They can be put on official notice when they receive a certified letter of your concerns, including a request for a response letter of their intent of action. You have a right to clean, healthy drinking water. Ultimately, it is your responsibility to assure that the quality of water you are receiving is at its best for consumption.

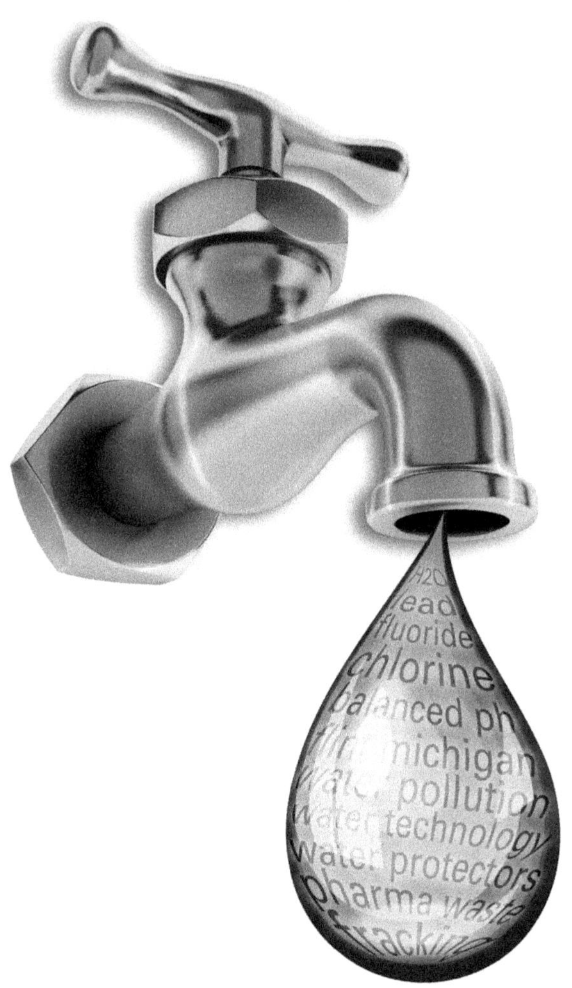

H2O
lead
fluoride
chlorine
balanced ph
flint michigan
water pollution
water technology
water protectors
pharma waste
fracking

CHAPTER 16

REMEDIATION IDEAS FOR AT HOME

Source: Homeowners look for ways to improve the quality of their tap water as they address issues concerning water sources that have been affected by pollution.

Advances in water filtration technology have drastically improved, allowing for more affordable options from which home owners may choose. These provide a variety of solutions to resolve these issues.

As increasing numbers of municipalities continue to face the challenges of outside pollution sources entering public water supplies. more home owners are now taking personal responsibility to acquire clean drinking water. They are educating themselves in areas of science and green technology to assure they have healthy, clean drinking water for their households and their families. Cities like Flint, Michigan, are still struggling with aging water delivery systems and decaying infrastructure, while also trying to source drinking water from supplies less influenced by pollution.

Even private wells may be affected by outside influences that have made their way into the well water supply deep in the ground. Some private wells are in areas where heavy minerals and metals are naturally found, resulting in hard water which will require filtration.

Concerns about fracking for oil and natural gas have increased the need to filter underground water sources. Home owners search for the best options that will insure better water quality for their personal consumption.

Water treatment systems can improve the quality of water supplies and reduce the hazards created by bacteria, chemical pollutants, and toxic substances. Before a system for the home is purchased, the water should be tested to determine the best option to rid the water of pollutants.

No two homes are the same. Some homes, even if they are next door, can differ in the issues surrounding water contamination and purification. A home's infrastructure, piping, well, water basin, tanks, coils, etc. can also affect water quality.

The most common water treatment systems utilized for the home are disinfection practices such as chlorination, ultraviolet light and radio frequency. Others are filtration using carbon filters and disposable cartridges, reverse osmosis, distillation, and ion exchanges in water softener units. There are additional methods that can be instituted for purifying a water supply in the home. The range varies from practices that cost little or no money to sophisticated systems that can cost thousands of dollars.

Disinfection systems are designed to kill and remove harmful bacteria, viruses and other agents which cause illness and disease from the water supplies.

Four disinfection methods include chlorination, treating water with ultraviolet light, radio frequency, and pasteurizing. Water can be disinfected by boiling it.

The oldest and most common method of disinfection is chlorination. An automated pump injects chlorine in small amounts into the water supply. Chlorine is an oxidizing agent that kills most bacteria and viruses. Using chlorine must be done with caution. Chlorine reacts to heavy metals, so additional filters with disposable cartridges are recommended. Chlorine is harmful to humans, plants and animals. Hence it is not the healthiest option but sometimes worth the cost depending on the situation.

Pasteurization and boiling water are cost effective ways to address cleaning water supplies, although both can be time consuming. Both practices destroy bacteria by heating the water to a high temperature. Boiled water has a flat taste since the oxygen and carbon dioxide have been removed.

Most municipalities that experience a disruption in service when water pipe infrastructure is serviced, recommend boiling water before usage. This is meant as a short term remedy only.

Ultraviolet light sterilization uses a system of low-pressure mercury lamps to produce rays of ultraviolet light which then projects its radiant heat to the targeted source of treatment. This process kills bacteria but is less effective on viruses and some other living organisms. Lamps require replacement because they degrade over time and their effectiveness decreases.

Radio frequency works in a similar fashion. Radio frequency of light pulses of electrical current charge pipes and tubes, decreasing water scale. An additional filter system is needed to remove granular material left after the UV light or radio frequency processes.

There are several types of filters available for water treatment. Water test results will indicate the filtration system that will be most effective. Mechanical filters are designed to remove sand, dirt, grit, salt, clay, and organic matter.

These systems are usually used with other water treatment options because mechanical filters do not address bacteria and virus cultures living in tainted water supplies. These filters are made from a host of materials including paper, fabric, ceramic, or metal screening materials, and need to be serviced on a regular basis as granular material is collect on them.

Active carbon filters soak up water impurities into the filter cartridge. These filters are used to remove chlorine chemical residue, odors and agents that influence taste. Some advanced carbon filters are designed to remove radon gas. These filters can be highly effective in dealing with basic water treatment contaminates but they are unable to treat highly polluted water sources.

These filters need to be integrated into the home using other types of water treatment. It may be necessary to find a healthier clean drinking water source. These filters lose their ability to treat water effectively as impurities are collected, and must be changed when they no longer filter adequately.

Oxidizing filters remove iron, manganese, and sulfur. This is an alternative to water softener treatment systems. To treat acidic water supplies, naturalizing filters are a viable option. This filtration system uses broken limestone chips as the catalyst to remove lead, copper, and other toxic heavy metals that leach into water from aging water infrastructure. This is one contributor to Flint, Michigan's dilemma because the aging infrastructure has been neglected. Other cities are experiencing similar challenges.

Another option for home water treatment is reverse osmosis. This process includes pressurizing and forcing water through a filtering membrane which removes 80-90% of contaminate impurities and granular material.

Mechanical and carbon filters utilize a reverse osmosis system. The filters remove granular material, impurities, and contaminates before the water passes through the membrane. These systems are costly. However, they are recommended for cooking and food preparation and must be checked on a regular basis for form and functionality.

Distillation is the process of boiling water, collecting the steam and then cooling the steam back to water. This process removes all minerals, impurities and bacteria as the unwanted agents are left behind. This is a relatively slow process. Only five to ten gallons of water are distilled at a time. Five gallons of regular unfiltered water from the faucet will produce just one gallon of distilled water. Stills require more maintenance than other systems and can be costly.

Ion exchangers are water softener systems. Most homes supplied by private well water have an issue with hard water. The mineral content makes the water very course. Iron, calcium and magnesium in excessive amounts result in hard water.

These minerals can wreak havoc on copper pipes, coils, and faucets because they react with metal. In the process of an ion exchanger, water is pumped through a tank which is treated with salt crystals. These dissolve the minerals. The water then passes through a series of filters to extract the impurities and smaller granular materials. These are the most common systems found in homes with private wells.

Before purchasing any system, several factors should be considered. It may be cheaper to rent or buy a system. The life span and return of investment of each system should be considered as well. Consumer ratings on these systems should be investigated. Some water treatment systems are more popular than others depending on the geographic area. Systems should be installed by a professional because they involve tying into new or existing plumbing and/or electrical systems. Local town permits may be required when installing a water treatment remediation system.

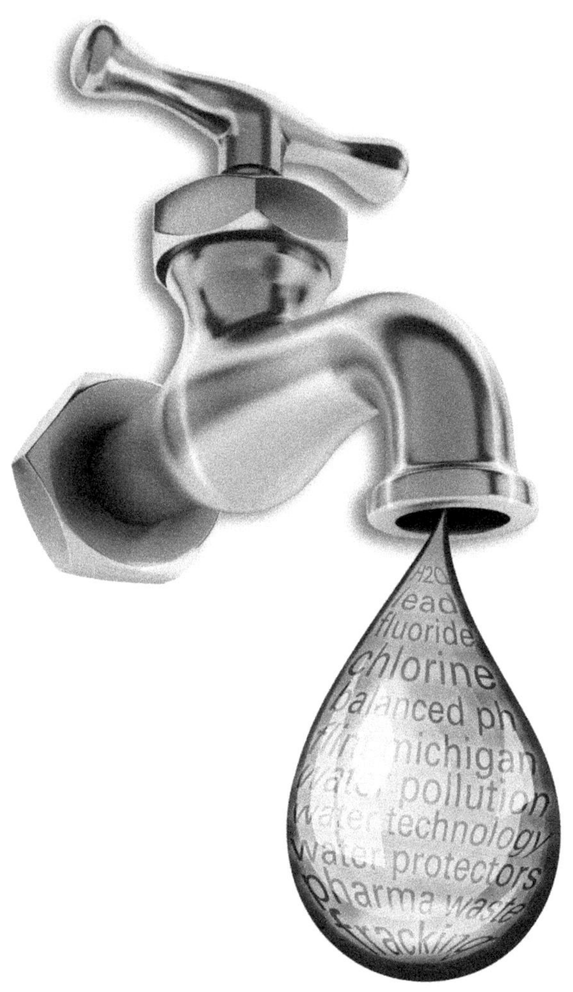

H2O
lead
fluoride
chlorine
balanced ph
michigan
water pollution
water technology
water protectors
pharma waste
fracking

CHAPTER 17

WATER PRESERVATION AND CONSERVATION TIPS FOR USE AT HOME

Source: Efforts are being made to conserve and protect our most important natural resource, water. This is occurring on local, state and federal government levels. Scientists and industrial professionals are used as consultants. Taking personal responsibility is paramount, as every citizen plays a vital role in protecting and conserving clean, fresh drinking water and ensuring that future generations will have access to this precious commodity. Here we address a few practices that can be used in the home to assist in conservation.

Who would have imagined fifty years ago we would be purchasing most of the drinking water we consume at our local grocery store, convenience store or corner market. In addition, clean water is needed for cleaning, laundry, cooking, baths, showers, irrigation, gardens, lawns, and for washing the car.

Throughout the home, we can diminish the ways we waste water. Whether you have a private well or pay for public water, these conservation tips should be considered.

Replace or repair leaking faucets, as every drip matters. Though we may not think of each drip as significant, water wasted adds up to dollars and cents over time.

According to the US Geological Survey, 15,140 drips equal one gallon of water (give or take a drip). Four thousand drips equal one liter of water. The average home drips one liter per day or 104 gallons per year. This is based on a home with three leaking faucets. The larger the home, the more bathrooms it has, the larger the loss could be. One solution is to replace faucets and showerheads with more efficient ones.

Leaking pipes in walls and basements are not as noticeable as the leaking faucets you see. Check all plumbing connections and drain pipes. Repair leaking pipes and replace old and corroded ones.

Check for leaking toilets or worn out toilet bowl floats. A toilet float that is not working properly may run for hours, causing many gallons of clean water to flow down the drain.

The wax seal around the bottom of the toilet bowl should be kept in good repair.

Only full loads of laundry should be run. Half loads use almost the same amount of water as full loads and take about the same amount of time to complete. The same goes for the dishwasher.

When attending to personal grooming needs, one should shut off the water after wetting a toothbrush until it is time to rinse. Water should not run while shaving. Much water flows from faucet to drain in these brief few minutes of usage.

Lawns and gardens can be demanding on water supplies. Water the lawn only when it is needed. To avoid using drinking water for watering flower beds, garden, or lawn, install rain barrels under the downspouts of gutters. Collect the run-off water from the roof during rain storms to be used for gardening. A small pump in the bottom of the barrel and a hose can eliminate the need to scoop out the water with a bucket.

When washing a car, the hose should not run continually. Rinse the vehicle initially, then shut the water off while soaping and scrubbing off tar and bug stains. Only when it is time to rinse off the soap should the water be turned on. A car wash that recycles water is also an option.

Technology can monitor and control your water usage. Rain gauges integrated into your sprinkler-irrigation system will automatically shut down watering systems when enough water is present. Toilet tank bags are designed to take up space in the toilet tank, so less water is used when the tank refills. Water flow valves are an inexpensive way to restrict the amount of water needed to flow through pipes to faucets. They are also a second line of defense to a leaking faucet. Energy efficient appliances, such as washing machines and dish washers, are a wise choice.

It is important to be mindful of what we put down the drain. Everything allowed down the drain or introduced into the eco-system will eventually enter our water supply. Sending expired or unused pharmaceutical prescription drugs down the toilet is a practice from the past that is now being discouraged. Today there are drop off points at local waste disposal stations, recycling centers, and some police stations that accept unused or expired medications.

Prescription drugs are chemical compounds not natural to lakes, rivers, streams, or groundwater. As prescription drugs dissolve in water, the chemicals make their way into fish, plants, and other aquatic wildlife. Pharma chemicals are very difficult to filter because they become trace chemicals.

Paint, oil, antifreeze, pesticides, or other harmful chemical agents should not be dumped down the drain. These chemicals may affect an entire clean water supply. Most municipal recycling centers will accept chemicals, oils and left over paint at their facilities. They have specific practices for managing the waste. If there is a significant amount of hazardous chemicals, a service will collect them for a fee.

Old cars should not be left to rot or decay on lawns, in fields, or in the woods. As time goes by, oxygen and water begin to turn the metal body and its metal parts into rust. Oil pans and gas tanks may rust as well. Even the smallest pin hole can result in leakage of gas and oil into ground water sources. Before storing old vehicles, all oils, fuels, and fluids should be drained completely.

Organic fertilizers and pesticides are more environmentally friendly than hard chemical products. Petro based chemical fertilizers and pesticides can wreak havoc on neighboring water supplies and ground water. Most lake communities have banned the use of fertilizers and pesticides because the run off of these chemicals into nearby lakes has caused significant algae and seaweed growth. The result is a decline in the quality of life for boaters, fishermen, and aquatic life.

When cleaning yards in the spring or fall, leaves should not be blown into drains or local waterways. Catch basin areas and gullies installed for flood control should not be polluted, even with natural garbage. These areas are created to carry off sediment, waste water, and run-off to their final destination. Leaves, sticks, and grass can clog drainage systems and act as a collection point for man-made garbage. This may eventually sink to the bottom of these drains or gullies or be carried off to lakes, streams, and other waterways. An overabundance of natural garbage can create an imbalance of the eco-system.

Pet fish or other pets should not be deposited into natural waterways. When people need to dispose of a live animal, such as a pet fish, snake, or turtle, they may want to release them into the local wild. This is a form of pollution known as pet pollution. When a species of fish or reptile is introduced into an eco-system not native to that species, it changes the entire chemistry of that eco-system. It has been discovered that a common practice is for people to dump their koi fish into a local river or stream. The koi can take over the natural setting as their own. This can have devastating effects on other species of fish that rely on the ecosystem in these waters they call home.

Koi compete for the same plankton, small insects, and small minnows that many native fish need to survive. An example of this occurred at a lake in Boulder, Colorado. This lake was a source of clean, fresh drinking water. The koi changed the chemistry of the water. The waste of the koi was very acidic and toxic to other fish. This affected the quality of the water for drinking purposes.

It is everyone's responsibility to protect and preserve our water sources. The uncontaminated drinking water for future generations depends on the choices we make today.

APPENDIX:

CITED RESOURCES

(In order of appearance and usage)

1. *"Public Supply Water Use,"* published by U.S. Geological Survey; Released, March 2004, Revised, February 2005. Written by Susan S. Hutson, Nancy L. Barber, Joan F. Kenny, Kristin S. Linsey, Deborah S. Lumia, and Molly A. Maupin

2., *"Water for a Sustainable World"*, UN World Water Development Report 2015; published by United Nations Educational, Scientific and Cultural Organization (UNESCO); on behalf of the United Nations World Water Assessment Program

3. *"Agency Superfund National Priorities List,"* published by United States Environmental Protection hosted at www.epa.gov/superfund/nationa-priorities-list-npl-states#NJ, updated on November, 29, 2016

4. *"Is New Jersey Really Green,"* article written by Samuel K. Burlum, Investigative Reporter, published March, 23, 2015, on www.SamBurlum.com

5. *"Ringwood is not the only trouble spot,"* article written by Jan Barry, staff writer, The Record, August 7, 2009

6. *"Final Report,"* published by the Flint Water Advisory Task Force; released March 2016; Commissioned by the Office of Governor Rick Snyder State of Michigan

7. *"California Drought Crop Sectors,"* published by United States Department of Agriculture Economic Research Service; last updated, Friday, February 03, 2017; located at https://www.ers.usda.gov/topics/in-the-news/california-drought-farm-and-food-impacts/california-drought-crop-sectors.aspx

8. *"Desalination,"* updated on February 25, 2017; page found at Wikipedia, https://en.wikipedia.org/wiki/Desalination

9. *"Sales of leading bottled still water brands in the United States 2016,"* published on May 15, 2016; by Statista found at www.Statista.com

10. *"Drinking-Water Fact Sheet,"* published by the World Health Organization; reviewed and released on November 2016

11. *"50 Reasons to Oppose Fluoridation",* by Dr. Paul Connett, PhD; updated on Sept. 2012; posted on FluorideAlert.Org

12. *"Fluoride in Drinking Water,"* Committee on Fluoride in Drinking Water, Board on Environmental Studies and Toxicology, Division on Earth and Life Studies, National Research Council; 2006

13. *"Chlorination, Cholorination by-product, and cancer: a meta-analysis,"* American Journal of Public Health July 1992; written by RD Morris, AM Audet, IF Angelillo, TC Chalmers, and F Mosteller

14. *"Pharmaceuticals Found in Drinking Water,"* by Jeff Donn, Martha Mendoza and Justin Pritchard, Associated Press; Investigation and Study; March 2006

15. *"USGS Groundwater Information Pages,"* published by U.S. Geological Survey; https://water.usgs.gov/ogw/

16. *"Where Does the Best Water Come From?"* written by Samuel K. Burlum, Investigative Reporter; published July 15, 2016; on www.H2OEnergyFlow.com

17. *"The purest water in the world?"* written by Fraser Los, Canadian Geographic Magazine; published June 1, 2011

18. *"Water, an Endangered Global Resource,"* written by Richard Mills, Ahead of the Heard; Report published on Aheadoftheheard.com

19. *"America's Most Endangered Rivers of 2015,"* written by Amy Kober, American Rivers, in Water Currents; April 7, 2015; supported by National Geographic

20. *"Our Drinkable Water Supply is Vanishing,"* written by Tara Lohan, AlterNet.org; October 10, 2007

21. *"State of the Industry: Bottled Water in the US,"* Published report, December 2016, 11th Edition, available for purchase

22. *"World Water Day Report,"* by the World Health Organization, found at www.who.int/water_sanitation_health

23. *"Nutrition and Healthy Eating- Water: How much should you drink every day?"* Published by the Mayo Clinic Staff; September 5, 2015

24. *"Water: the Single Most Important Element for Your Health,"* Dr. Joseph Mercola interviews Dr. Gerald Pollack, January 29, 2011; syndicated on You Tube

25. *"The Effects of Toxic Metals,"* written by Dr. Edward Group, Global Healing Center; published on March 18, 2013

26. *"How Water Works,"* by Shanna Freeman; posted on HowStuffWorks.com; October 18, 2007,

27. *"A Special Report: The Chemistry of Water,"* by the National Science Foundation, located within the www. nsdl.org website

28. *"Industrial Water Use: Estimated Use of Water in the United States in 2000,"* written by Susan S. Hutson, Nancy L. Barber, Joan F. Kenny, Kristin S. Linsey, Deborah S. Lumia, and Molly A. Maupin, US Geological Survey; updated Feb. 2005

29. *"What the Frack?"* written by Samuel K. Burlum, Investigative Reporter; published May, 23, 2014; The Alternative Press.com (now known as TapInto.com)

30. *"Analysis: NJ environmentalist optimistic about 2017,"* written by Scott Fallon, Staff Writer; North Jersey.com; published December 28, 2016

31. *"Demonstration calls for Ban on Fracking in the Delaware River Shed,"* written by David Pringle, Press Release, February 15, 2017; by Clean Water Action

32. *"New Jersey Senate Passes Fracking Waste Ban,"* written by Brandon Baker, May 12, 2014; EcoWatch.com

33. *"Standing Rock Protest: This is only the beginning,"* written by Rebecca Solnit, The Guardian; September 12, 2016

34. *"Here's What You Should Know about the Dakota Pipeline Protest,"* written by Joseph Erbentraut, Huffington Post; posted November 2, 2016; Updated Jan. 15, 2017

35. *"Not All the Standing Rock Sioux are protesting the pipeline,"* written by Jessica Ravitz, CNN, posted November 3, 2016

36. *"Euphrates-Tigris Basin Facts,"* posted by the Food and Agriculture Organization, of the United Nations, full report at: http://www.fao.org/nr/water/aquastat/basins/euphrates-tigris/Euphrates.tigris-CP_eng.pdf

37. *"The Mesopotamian Marshlands; The Demise of an Ecosystem,"* Division of Early Warning And Assessment Technical Report, United Nations Environmental Program; prepared by Hassan Partow; published 2001

38. *"Minnesota Senate moves to clarify buffers, part of new water quality law,"* written by Don Davis, Forum News Service, and posted on Twin Cities/Pioneer Press; published April 14, 2016

39. *"Buffer bull passes, sent to Gov. Mark Dayton for Signature,"* written by J. Patrick Coolican, Star Tribune, April 21, 2016

40. *"Healthy Soils Imitative,"* posted by Califionia Climate and Agriculture Network, also known as CalCAN on their site 2016; http://calclimateag.org/healthysoils/

41. *"Florida Passes Statewide Water and Natural Resources Policy,"* by Sunshine State News, January 13, 2016

42. *"Florida Senate Bill, SB 552; 2016,"* written by Florida State Senator Dean, posted by the Florida State Senate, at https://www.flsenate.gov/Session/Bill/2016/0552/BillText/Filed/PDF

43. *"New Water Quality Standards for the State of Vermont,"* found at published report and rulemaking; Vermont Dept. of Environmental Conservation; http://dec.vermont.gov/sites/dec/files/documents/wsmd_water_quality_standards_2016.pdf

44. *"Water Resources Development Act of 2016,"* Sponsored by Sen. James Inholfe, R-OK, view total bill, updates, and progress at: https://www.congress.gov/bill/114th-congress/senate-bill/2848

45. *"Water Resources Development Act of 2016,"* Sponsored by Rep. Bill Shuster, R-PA-9; view total bill, update and progress at: https://www.congress.gov/bill/114th-congress/house-bill/5303

46. *"World Bank's New Environmental and Social Framework is a Huge Step Backward for Human*

Rights," written by Upasana Khatri, Earth Rights International, August, 17, 2017, Earth Rights.org

47. *"World Bank Board Approves New Environmental and Social Framework,"* Press Release posted by the World Bank, August 4, 2016; WorldBank.org

48. *"Drinking Water Regulatory Information,"* published by the US EPA, with additional resources at their webpage: https://www.epa.gov/dwreginfo/drinking-water-regulatory-information

49. *"New Technology Aimed at Reducing Water Usage,"* written by Samuel K. Burlum, Investigative Reporter, published on H2OEnergyFlow.com, Jan. 15, 2017

50. *"Drip Accumulator: How much water does a leaking faucet waste?"* published by the US Geological Survey, updated on December 2, 2016; posted at webpage: https://water.usgs.gov/edu/dripcalculator.html

51. *"Methods for Testing the Quality of Water At Home,"* written by Samuel K. Burlum, Investigative Reporter, published on H2OEnergyFlow.com, October 30, 2016

52. *"Water Quality & Testing,"* by the Centers for Disease Control and Prevention; updated April 10,

2009; available at: https://www.cdc.gov/healthywater/
drinking/public/water_quality.html

53. ***"Why Save Water,"*** by the US EPA, early education
for kids about water, at: https://www3.epa.gov/
watersense/kids/whysave.html

APPENDIX:

GLOSSARY

Acidic: having the properties of an acid, or containing acid; having a pH below 7. Acidic water can absorb toxins like mercury.

Alkaline: in drinking water, references the pH level, generally a pH of 8 or 9.

Aquifer: The saturated zone beneath the water table; underground layer of water-bearing permeable rock, rock fractures or unconsolidated materials (gravel, sand, or silt) from which groundwater can be extracted using a water well.

Artesian well: a well that doesn't require a pump to bring water to the surface; wells that are drilled into aquifers.

BPA free: Bisphenol A (BPA) is an organic synthetic compound used to produce reusable plastic products.

Due to evidence that suggests negative health effects of BPA, products such as recycled plastic water bottles may be manufactured "BPA free," meaning without BPA included in the manufacturing of the product.

Brownfields: a former industrial or commercial site that may have hazardous substances, pollutants or contaminants present.

Climate change: a change in global or regional climate patterns.

Chlorination: the process of adding chlorine or hypochlorite to water to kill certain bacteria as well as other microbes in tap water.

C40 Cities Climate Leadership Group: a network of the world's megacities committed to addressing climate change.

De-ionized: when water has had almost all of its mineral ions removed; also known as demineralized water.

Distilled: water that has had many of its impurities removed through distillation, involving boiling the water, then condensing the steam into a clean container.

Eco-system: a biological community of interacting organisms and their physical environment; a system including all living things in a given area, which interact with each other as well as non-living things.

Environmental justice: the fair treatment and purposeful involvement of all people regardless of race, color, national origin, or income with respect to the development, implementation, and enforcement of environmental laws, regulations, and policies.

Filtration: any process, mechanical, physical or biological that separates solids from fluids (liquids or gases) by adding a medium through which only the fluid can pass.

Fluoridation: the process where a controlled amount of fluoride is added to a public water supply for the purpose of reducing tooth decay.

Global warming: term used to describe a gradual increase in the average temperature of the Earth's atmosphere and its oceans, with the belief that the Earth's climate may be permanently changed.

Hydro-fracking: hydraulic fracturing; a technique where large amounts of water are combined with smaller amounts of sand and chemicals, and then pumped under high pressure into a drilled gas well.

Monotonic: a function or quantity varying in such a way that it either never decreases or never increases; unchanging.

MTBE free: Methyl tert-butyl ether (MTBE) is a gasoline additive used as an oxygenate and to raise the octane number. MTBE has been found to pollute groundwater resulting from gasoline spills.

MUA (municipal utilities authority): municipalities providing wastewater collection and treatment services as well as solid waste and recycling services in order to protect the public safety, welfare, and health of residents within its assigned areas.

Natural: existing in or caused by nature; not made or caused by humankind.

Osmosis: a process by which molecules of a solvent tend to pass through a semipermeable membrane from a less concentrated solution into a more concentrated one, thus equalizing the concentrations on each side of the membrane.

Pasteurization: the process of using heat to kill pathogenic bacteria in a liquid or in food to make the food safe to eat.

Parts per million (ppm): usually describing the concentration of something in water or soil. One ppm is equivalent to 1 milligram of something per liter of water (mg/l) or 1 milligram of something per kilogram of soil (mg/kg).

PCB (polychlorinated biphenyls): an organic chlorine compound that is man-made, consisting of carbon, hydrogen and chlorine atoms. PCBs vary in toxicity level and in consistency from thin, light-colored liquids to yellow or black waxy solids.

Permafrost: soil, rock or sediment that is frozen for more than two consecutive years.

Pollution: the presence in or introduction into the environment of a substance or thing that has harmful or poisonous effects.

Purification: the removal of contaminants from something; with water, the process removes harmful chemicals, biological contaminants, suspended solids and gases from contaminated water with the intent to produce water fit for a specific use.

pH: pH (potential of hydrogen) is a numeric scale used to specify the acidity or basicity of an aqueous solution.

Runoff: the draining away of water (or substances carried in it) from the surface of an area of land, a building or structure, etc.

Spring water: water from a spring, as opposed to river water or rainwater.

Sustainable: the property of biological systems to remain diverse and productive indefinitely.

Trace minerals: minerals needed for human consumption and health that are organic in matter and cannot be destroyed by cooking or heat. These include Copper, Chromium, Fluoride, Iodine, Iron, Molybdenum, Manganese, Selenium, and Zinc.

ABOUT THE AUTHOR

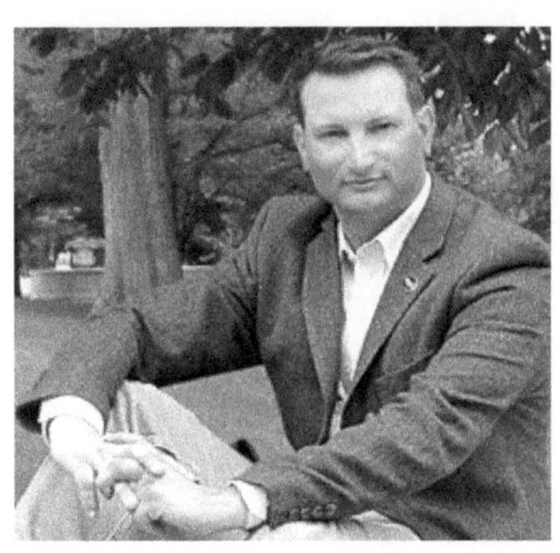

Samuel K. Burlum is a career entrepreneur, author and investigative reporter, who's career dates back to 1992 when he founded his first business. Burlum's area of expertise is within the green industry, including green technology, green related consumer products, and public policy relating to environmental concerns.

Mr. Burlum holds an Associate's Degree in Applied Sciences, having majored in Business Management while attending Berkeley College, Woodland Park, NJ.

Currently Mr. Burlum is the CEO and President of Extreme Energy Solutions, Inc., a green tech company which brings to the market green, eco-friendly consumer products and emissions reduction technology for the automotive and transportation industry.

Burlum is a consultant for small to medium businesses, specializing in providing them guidance and expertise in the areas of strategic business planning, business development, supply chain management, and systems integration.

He is also the author of "The Green Lane," which is the compilation of syndicated articles and a column that reports on public policy debates and concerns focusing on small businesses and environmental justice.

His contributions to public policy include formally testifying at hearings related to air and water quality. Mr. Burlum also provided content for consideration with regards to new legislation dealing with environmental compliance, small business research and development, technology, and tax code reform.

Burlum has been recognized by the World Green Energy Symposium, being awarded the 2013 NOVA Award on behalf of Extreme Energy Solutions, for their contributions in the field of green technology; addressing the issue of toxic harmful vehicle emissions while increasing engine efficiency.

He also was recognized by the People of Distinction Humanitarian Foundation and named as one of their 2014 Unsung Hero Award recipients.

The Passaic Valley FOP 181 also recognized Burlum and his company in the field of environmentally friendly products and services, naming his business Company of the Year in 2013, 2015, and 2016; while also naming Burlum a leader in the community.

He has been featured on media venues such as *Today in America* with Terry Bradshaw, and Cablevision's *Neighborhood Journal*, as well as in *Natural Awakenings* Magazine.

Samuel Burlum currently resides in scenic Sussex County, New Jersey, not far from his home town of West Milford, New Jersey.

For more information, you can reach Mr. Burlum by visiting his website at:

www.SamBurlum.com

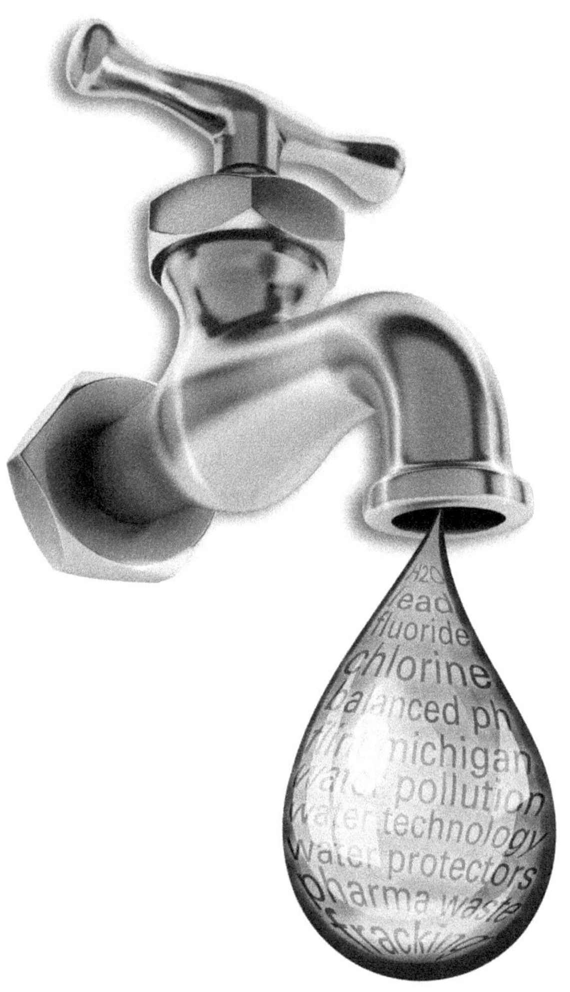

H2O
lead
fluoride
chlorine
balanced ph
flint michigan
water pollution
water technology
water protectors
pharma waste
fracking

OTHER BOOKS BY SAMUEL K. BURLUM:

"LIFE IN THE GREEN LANE; IN PURSUIT OF THE AMERICAN DREAM"

Based on a true story...

"Life in the Green Lane; in Pursuit of the American Dream," is based on a true story, written by Samuel K. Burlum; explaining the journey and experiences of a group of individuals that participated in one of the largest open source research projects in postmodern times; responsible for spurring off the green technology revolution in the field of fuel economy.

Led by a small group of people with a vision, they would take on the responsibility of legitimizing a movement into an industry segment within the automotive and green tech sector; sharing their challenges and trials along the way.

When it is discovered that the controversial Hydro Assist Fuel Cell can beyond deliver upon early expectations, in specific applications, it is met with great resistance from media, government, and industry skeptics.

"Life in the Green Lane- in Pursuit of the American Dream," is a true David versus Goliath story, where Samuel K. Burlum tells his side of the story regarding the series of events on how one group of individuals became the trend setters in taking an obscure technology, and launching it main stream.

Burlum shares the full details behind the science of fuel economy, and how he and his team deployed the Smart Emissions Reducer technology into the market. He also provides a full account of trials, challenges, and behind the scenes battles he, his team, and his company had to overcome in bringing this innovation to market.

ORDER ONLINE TODAY:

https://www.indiegogo.com/projects/life-in-the-green-lane-based-on-a-true-story-entrepreneurship#/

http://samburlum.com/about-life-in-the-green-lane/

OR YOU CAN ORDER

"LIFE IN THE GREEN LANE,"

THROUGH THE MAIL BY USING THE FORM

ON THE NEXT PAGE...

ORDER FORM:

"LIFE IN THE GREEN LANE;
IN PURSUIT OF THE AMERICAN DREAM"

Written by Samuel K. Burlum

Complete the information below, and then select the items you wish to buy. Send this form & your check/money order payable to:

Sam Burlum, PO Box 730, Hewitt, NJ 07421

You should receive your order within 7 to 10 business days of us processing your payment and confirming your order. We thank you for your business in advance.

"LIFE IN THE GREEN LANE; IN PURSUIT OF THE AMERICAN DREAM"

Type of Book Copy	Cost Each	No. of Copies	Total
Soft Cover	$24.99		
Hard Cover	$39.99		
E-book Version on CD	$9.99		
	Total	Order:	$

Includes FREE Shipping & Handling Cost

Name: ____

Mailing Address: _______________________________________

City/State/Zip Code: _____________________________________

Phone/email: ____

ORDER FORM:

*** Order a Copy Today for A Friend ***

"THE RACE TO PROTECT OUR MOST IMPORTANT NATURAL RESOURCE"

Written by Samuel K. Burlum

Complete the information below, and then select the items you wish to buy. Send this form & your check/money order payable to:

Sam Burlum, PO Box 730, Hewitt, NJ 07421

You should receive your order within 7 to 10 business days of us processing your payment and confirming your order. We thank you for your business in advance.

"LIFE IN THE GREEN LANE; IN PURSUIT OF THE AMERICAN DREAM"

Type of Book Copy	Cost Each	No. of Copies	Total
Soft Cover	$14.99		
E-book Version on CD	$4.99		
	Total	Order:	$

Includes FREE Shipping & Handling Cost

Name: ____

Mailing Address: ______________________________________

City/State/Zip Code: ___________________________________

Phone/email: ____

FOR MORE INFORMATION:

For more information about the author, Samuel K. Burlum, or to subscribe to his monthly articles, sign up today at:

www.SamBurlum.com

You can also visit these other websites for more information about other eco-friendly green technology and products:

www.ExtremeEnergySolutions.net

www.SmartEmissionsReducer.com

www.ExtremeKleaner.com

www.H2OEnergyFlow.com

Or you can join Samuel K. Burlum and the affiliated products on Social Media:

 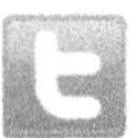 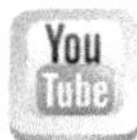